Critical Care Nephrology

Editor

Bruce A Molitoris, MD

Indiana University School of Medicine
Indianapolis, IN
USA

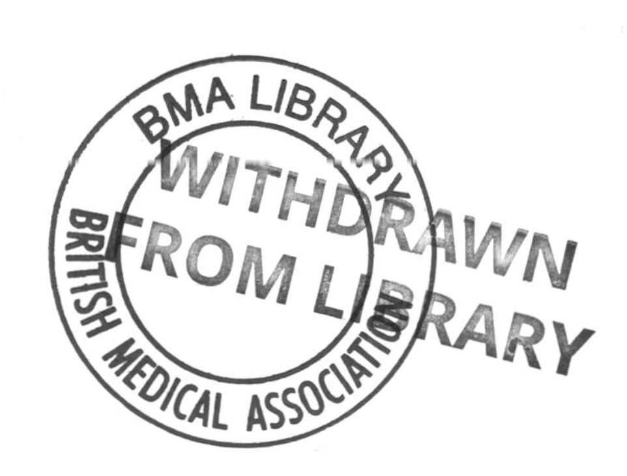

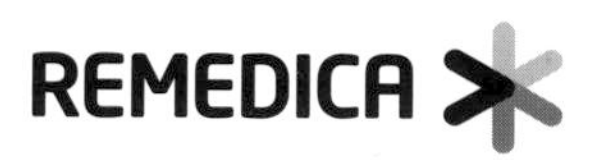

Editor

Bruce A Molitoris, MD

Professor of Medicine

Director of Nephrology

Director, Indiana Center for Biological Microscopy

Indiana University School of Medicine

1120 South Drive

Fesler Hall Room 115

Indianapolis, IN 46202

USA

Contributors

Matthew D Dollins, MD

Assistant Professor of Clinical Medicine

Nephrology Division

Indiana University School of Medicine

950 W. Walnut St.

R2 202

Indianapolis, IN 46202

USA

Michael A Kraus, MD

Associate Professor of Clinical Medicine

Nephrology Division

Indiana University School of Medicine

950 W. Walnut St.

R2 202

Indianapolis, IN 46202

USA

Richard N Hellman, MD

Associate Professor of Clinical Medicine

Nephrology Division

Indiana University School of Medicine

950 W. Walnut St.

R2 202

Indianapolis, IN 46202

USA

Edward Sha, MD

Nephrology Division

Indiana University School of Medicine

950 W. Walnut St.

R2 202

Indianapolis, IN 46202

USA

Critical Care Nephrology

Also available from Remedica
Kidney Transplantation
Editor: Donald E Hricik, University Hospitals of Cleveland, Cleveland, OH, USA
ISBN: 1 901346 49 8

Published by Remedica
32–38 Osnaburgh Street, London, NW1 3ND, UK
20 North Wacker Drive, Suite 1642, Chicago, IL 60606, USA

E-mail: info@remedicabooks.com
www.remedicabooks.com

Publisher: Andrew Ward
In-house editors: Tamsin White, James Griffin

Remedica is a member of the AS&K Media Partnership

ISBN 1 901346 66 8
British Library Cataloguing-in-Publication Data
A catalogue record for this book is available from the British Library

To the dedicated nephrology faculty at Indiana University School of Medicine, who provide an environment of broad-based learning and cooperation that maximally benefits patient care, research, and education.

Preface

Intensive care unit (ICU) nephrology is a rapidly emerging area of interest in medicine. Nephrologists have always participated in the care of critically ill patients, including those with electrolyte and acid–base disorders, volume disorders, hypertensive crisis, and acute renal failure. An increasing recognition of the overlap between critical care and nephrology, combined with recent advances in the understanding of acute renal failure and the application of renal replacement therapies, have served to highlight the important role the nephrologist plays in the ICU. This handbook has been written to provide all "students" of nephrology, irrespective of their level of training, with the latest knowledge regarding the care of critically ill patients. We have tried to provide all of the "essential" clinical, diagnostic, and therapeutic information that the reader will need, and have supplemented it with the most relevant physiology and pathophysiology. We hope you and your patients benefit from our efforts and that this book serves to refresh, clarify, and update your knowledge of critical care nephrology.

Bruce A Molitoris

Foreword

Homeostasis and health depend on intact renal function, and the acutely failing kidney adversely affects such diverse processes as volume regulation, cardiopulmonary function, electrolyte profile and balance, acid–base status, regulation of systemic hemodynamics, hemostasis, and assorted nutritional and metabolic profiles. These systemic and far-ranging effects of acute renal failure can impair the function of vital organs and contribute to heightened morbidity and mortality when acute renal failure develops in the critically ill patient. Critical illness itself, originating and evolving in major extrarenal systems and largely irrespective of the underlying cause, sets the stage for renal injury and significantly increases the risk for acute renal failure. The development of acute renal failure in the critically ill patient thus signifies a harmful feedback loop: acute renal failure is more likely to occur in these patients, and once present, acute renal failure decidedly worsens their overall prognosis. Consequently, one of the fundamental objectives in the management of patients in the intensive care setting is, essentially, a nephrologic one: the avoidance of risks and precipitants for acute renal failure, the prompt and effective management of renal insufficiency if it occurs, and the timely and judicious use of renal replacement therapy when renal failure is incipient or established.

The involvement of nephrology and nephrologists in the critical care unit, however, clearly extends beyond considerations of kidney failure. Disturbances in fluid and electrolyte status, acid–base disorders, the management of cardiac and liver failure, the control of systemic hypertension, and the management of intoxications are just some of the recognized areas wherein the expertise and involvement of the nephrologist add immeasurably to the management of patients in the intensive care setting. Additionally, an emerging interest in the application of dialytic techniques to treat conditions (such as the systemic inflammatory response syndrome) that are not necessarily related to renal failure or fluid/electrolyte/acid–base disorders could offer innovative opportunities for additional involvement by nephrologists. Thus, by providing understanding and expertise in these and related areas of nephrology, the nephrologist is an active participant in the critical care setting. Moreover, the long-established approach used in the practice of nephrology – that nephrologic diseases must be analyzed within the context of relevant systemic and extrarenal processes – concurs with the integrative approach generally employed in the management of critically ill patients.

Yet, there are very few texts that are dedicated to the practice of nephrology in the intensive care unit (ICU). *Critical Care Nephrology*, written by Dr Molitoris and faculty in the Nephrology Division at Indiana University School of Medicine, thus fills a void that exists among current texts in nephrology. While there are numerous complete texts in nephrology, as well as books devoted to fluids and electrolytes, acid–base disorders, dialysis, acute renal failure, and other areas, specific and concise coverage of nephrology in the ICU is clearly wanting. In addressing this need, this handbook comprehensively covers the topic under four main headings – stabilization, optimization, acute renal failure, and, finally, renal replacement therapy. Stabilization covers the topics of respiration and circulation, areas central to the care of the critically ill patient and a common interface for interaction among nephrologists, intensive care specialists, and other subspecialists. Optimization encompasses fluid and electrolyte disturbances, edema, disorders of acid–base and calcium–phosphate homeostasis, nutritional considerations, and issues related to transplant recipients. Acute renal failure, in all of its relevant aspects – including risk factors, etiology, clinical and laboratory assessment, prevention and management, outcomes and prognosis – is lucidly and extensively covered. The final section on renal replacement therapy discusses the various modalities that are currently available, their indications, prescriptions, advantages and potential drawbacks, and the vascular access employed for such renal replacement therapy. Importantly, this section points out that the rationale for such therapies has evolved from simply the prevention of uremia and its complications to continued and adequate support of the patient such that critical comorbid conditions can be more effectively treated.

This handbook succeeds, quite remarkably, at many levels, and thus will be greatly appreciated by a wide readership. The clarity with which the text is written, the ease with which understanding is imparted, and the comprehensiveness and completeness of the various chapters, in aggregate, make this handbook eminently suitable for the medical student, resident, and fellow in nephrology. The handbook provides information in a clear, concise, and logical manner, is accessible and portable, and includes appropriate tables and easy-to-follow diagrams. Additionally, by its rigor and depth, this handbook provides an outstanding review and *aide-mémoire* for the staff nephrologist, an appeal for whom is further heightened by the inclusion, where relevant, of new and important findings from recent studies, and a succinct listing of critical references. Finally, this handbook, by its collective virtues, provides excellent instruction for trainees and practitioners in other critical care disciplines who wish to acquire an understanding of critical care nephrology.

Dr Molitoris and his colleagues are to be highly commended for undertaking the demanding task of compiling a new and much needed text in critical care nephrology, and for the outstanding handbook that has emanated from their collective efforts. This invaluable handbook is highly recommended to trainees and practitioners in nephrology, and to anyone involved in critical care wishing a comprehension of relevant areas of nephrology. By providing this wonderful instruction in critical care nephrology and its practice, Dr Molitoris and his colleagues have ultimately served, and admirably so, the needs of patient care in this setting.

Karl A Nath
Professor of Medicine, Mayo Clinic College of Medicine, MN, USA

Contents

Section 1

Stabilization

Part 1: Airway and breathing

Part 2: Circulation

Part 1: Airway and breathing

Matthew D Dollins

Acute respiratory failure

Acute respiratory failure is defined as the inability of the respiratory system to meet the oxygenation, ventilation, or metabolic requirements of the patient. This may occur in a previously healthy person with pneumonia or pulmonary embolism, or complicating the course of a patient with chronic respiratory failure in the setting of pulmonary fibrosis and chronic obstructive pulmonary disease (COPD). Respiratory failure can be divided into two main types: hypoxemic respiratory failure (failure to maintain adequate oxygenation); and hypercapnic respiratory failure (inadequate ventilation with CO_2 retention) (see **Table 1**).

Hypoxemic respiratory failure

When treating a patient with hypoxemia, oxygen should be provided by the least invasive approach possible. If the hypoxemia is potentially rapidly reversible, such as with congestive heart failure (CHF) or hypoventilation secondary to narcotic overdose, intubation may be avoided. Patients who are hypoxemic and alert may benefit from a trial of noninvasive ventilation such as continuous positive airway pressure (CPAP) or bi-level positive airway pressure (BiPAP). Exacerbations of CHF and COPD have been treated successfully with these mechanisms. However, prolonged hypoxemia can have adverse effects on end-organ function, and should be avoided. When noninvasive methods fail, the patient is unable to protect their airway, or the patient is in severe respiratory distress, intubation should be performed.

Hypercapnic respiratory failure

Hypercapnic respiratory failure is most common in exacerbations of COPD and hypoventilation secondary to loss of consciousness. In a patient with a reduced level of consciousness that

Table 1. Causes of respiratory failure.

ARDS: acute respiratory distress syndrome; AV: arteriovenous; CNS: central nervous system; COPD: chronic obstructive pulmonary disease; OD: overdose; V/Q: ventilation/perfusion.

Hypoxemic respiratory failure		Hypercapnic respiratory failure		
V/Q mismatch	**Shunt**	**CNS**	**Muscle dysfunction**	**Mechanical**
Pulmonary embolism Asthma/COPD Interstitial lung disease	Pneumonia Pulmonary edema ARDS Lung collapse Pulmonary AV fistula Cardiac left to right shunt	Stroke Elimination of hypoxic drive Drug OD Intoxication Trauma with loss of consciousness	Guillain–Barré syndrome Myasthenia gravis Severe COPD/ asthma	Pneumothorax Flail chest

cannot be quickly corrected, intubation is mandatory. However, patients with COPD exacerbations may be able to improve with bronchodilator and corticosteroid treatment and may not require intubation.

There is no mandatory pCO_2 (partial pressure of CO_2) at which a patient should be intubated, as many patients have a baseline pCO_2 as high as 70 mm Hg. However, if an acute respiratory acidosis occurs, in addition to the falling pH potentially causing cellular damage, the worsening hypercapnia can make the patient somnolent, further reducing the respiratory drive and leading to a cycle of worsening respiratory acidosis. Those patients with somnolence, or worsening respiratory acidosis despite treatment, should be intubated and receive mechanical ventilation.

Noninvasive ventilation

In the last decade, there has been renewed interest in noninvasive positive pressure ventilation (NPPV) for patients with respiratory failure. NPPV techniques include CPAP and BiPAP, and have the advantage of shorter length of hospitalization and a lower rate of nosocomial pneumonia compared with invasive mechanical ventilation. Both modalities consist of a tight fitting nasal or full-face mask that must be carefully selected and applied to avoid air leaks, eye irritation, and nasal abrasion. The nasal mask is more prone to air leak, which can diminish its efficacy, and requires the patient to keep his/her mouth closed so as to avoid air leak. The full-face mask is becoming more popular due to the lesser chance of air leak, but cannot be used in the obtunded patient as vomiting could lead to massive aspiration while wearing the tight-fitting mask.

Appropriate patient selection is important; the patient should be awake, cooperative, able to initiate each breath, and without excessive respiratory secretions. Patients with hemodynamic instability, inability to protect their airway, or obtundation should not receive NPPV. An uncooperative patient who will not leave their mask on or a patient on whom an adequate seal cannot be maintained secondary to nasogastric tubes or facial hair should prompt consideration of endotracheal intubation.

Continuous positive airway pressure

CPAP allows constant airflow at a preset pressure. It has been used for many years to treat obstructive sleep apnea, acting as a stent for the upper airway and thus preventing obstruction during the relaxed state of sleep. However, it is not commonly used for acute respiratory failure other than CHF exacerbations, as it is not as effective in reducing the work of breathing as BiPAP.

Bi-level positive airway pressure

BiPAP utilizes two levels of pressure. It combines positive end-expiratory pressure (PEEP) with a higher level of inspiratory pressure support (PS). The inspiratory support is in synch with the patient's inspiratory effort and, in patients with COPD, it increases the tidal volume, which can help with removal of CO_2. PEEP is used to overcome dynamic

Table 2. Contraindications to noninvasive positive pressure ventilation.

GCS: Glasgow coma scale.

Adapted from [2].

Contraindications
Cardiac or respiratory arrest
Nonrespiratory organ failure – Severe encephalopathy (eg, GCS<10) – Severe upper gastrointestinal bleeding – Hemodynamic instability or unstable cardiac arrhythmia
Facial surgery, trauma, or deformity
Upper airway obstruction
Inability to cooperate or protect the airway
Inability to clear respiratory secretions
High risk for aspiration

hyperinflation (auto-PEEP). In patients with CHF exacerbations, the inspiratory positive pressure increases tidal volume and decreases the amount of work required for breathing, while the PEEP helps keep the flooded alveoli open and increases the reabsorption of alveolar edema. COPD and CHF are the primary indications for BiPAP, although one study of 27 patients showed a higher rate of myocardial infarction in patients with cardiogenic pulmonary edema treated with BiPAP compared to CPAP [1]. Relatively stable patients with acute lung injury (ALI), severely immunosuppressed patients who are at high risk of ventilator-associated pneumonia, and patients with a "do not intubate" order may benefit from BiPAP. Contraindications to noninvasive ventilation are listed in **Table 2.**

When initiating BiPAP, low levels of PS and PEEP should be selected initially, and the mask should be placed gently over the patient's face to allow the patient to become accustomed to the positive pressure. Once the patient is used to the positive pressure, the mask can be secured, and the level of PS increased. Indications that an adequate amount of PS is being used include less labored breathing (decreased accessory muscle use, decreased respiratory rate [RR], and increased tidal volume), improved oxygenation, and improved arterial blood gases. Initial BiPAP settings are typically an inspiratory pressure of 8–10 mm Hg with a PEEP of 5 mm Hg. The inspiratory pressure can be increased to a maximum of 30 mm Hg. Patients placed on noninvasive ventilation need to be carefully monitored to ensure that they are benefiting from this mode of ventilation. Patients who deteriorate, are intolerant, or become obtunded should undergo endotracheal intubation.

Placing an artificial airway

The primary concern in treating a patient with respiratory distress or failure is securing the airway. It is preferable to make an assessment of the patient's respiratory status early in the course of their illness and, if intubation is deemed necessary, to perform this when time can be taken to gather the appropriate equipment and perform a smooth intubation, as emergency intubations are associated with a higher failure rate and morbidity. Endotracheal intubation is indicated to provide mechanical ventilation to patients with impending or established respiratory failure, and to provide airway protection to patients who are at risk for aspiration (eg, patients with mental status changes) or who have excessive

Table 3. Indications for intubation.

BiPAP: bi-level positive airway pressure; COPD: chronic obstructive pulmonary disease; PaO_2: partial pressure of O_2 in arterial blood.

Indications for intubation
Inability to protect airway
Severe head injury
High spinal cord trauma
Copious thick respiratory secretions
Acute exacerbation of COPD with progressive respiratory acidosis that has any of the following: - failed BiPAP - hemodynamic instability - abnormalities of the face preventing BiPAP use - severe somnolence
Neuromuscular disease causing respiratory failure with any of the following: - respiratory acidosis - forced vital capacity <10–15 mL/kg - progressive decline in maximal inspiratory pressure to <20–30 cm H_2O
Acute hypoxemic respiratory failure (PaO_2 <60) despite high flow oxygen via face mask with any of the following: - failed BiPAP - hemodynamic instability - severe somnolence - profound agitation

tracheobronchial secretions (see **Table 3**). If there is any concern that the patient may not be able to protect his/her airway, they should be intubated to prevent a potentially catastrophic aspiration pneumonitis or pneumonia.

Orotracheal intubation

Once the decision has been made to intubate a patient, the necessary equipment should be placed within easy reach of the physician performing thc intubation (see **Table 4**). The first approach is usually orotracheal intubation, as this carries less risk of infection than the nasotracheal route [3]. Failure to establish an airway can occur in any setting and leads to severe anxiety for the physician, as well as increased morbidity and mortality for the patient. Therefore, anyone who is responsible for intubating patients should be comfortable with more than one technique. Alternate methods include nasotracheal intubation (which may be better tolerated in the conscious patient), intubating laryngeal mask airway, transtracheal jet ventilation, or placement of a surgical airway.

Sedation for intubation

Pharmacologic agents are commonly used to increase the ease and success of intubation. Failure to place an airway after sedation or paralysis can lead to severe hypoxia and death if the patient cannot be ventilated. Therefore, the physician performing the intubation should have a degree of confidence in the technique and, if there is a concern that an airway may be difficult, either the patient should not be paralyzed, or alternative airway or physician backup should be made available.

"Rapid sequence intubation" is the rapid administration of an induction agent, followed by administration of a paralytic. Patients in cardiac arrest, in a coma, or those with no response

Table 4. Items required to perform an intubation.

Items
Laryngoscope
Laryngoscope blades
Endotracheal tube
Ambu bag with CO_2 detector
Oropharyngeal airway
Suction catheter
Sedatives/paralytics
Cardiac monitoring
Pulse oximeter

to insertion of the laryngoscope do not need to be medicated. If the likelihood of success is low, either due to the patient's anatomy or inability to open the mouth, these drugs should not be given.

Suitable induction agents include pentothal, etomidate, propofol, midazolam, or lorazepam. Pentothal has a rapid onset of action and can blunt the sympathetic response to laryngoscopy and intubation, but can cause peripheral vasodilatation. Etomidate lacks negative inotropic effects, but can cause vasodilation when given at a full dose, as well as myoclonic jerks on induction, nausea, and suppression of adrenal cortisol production. Propofol may reduce cerebral perfusion pressure and should not be used in a patient with increased intracranial pressure. Midazolam has a shorter half-life than lorazepam, and for this reason is the benzodiazepine of choice for intubation.

Pentothal, etomidate, and propofol have a rapid onset of action (within 10–15 seconds). If prescription of paralytics is planned, they can be given before the fast acting induction drugs because the paralytics have a slower onset of action. However, the benzodiazepines have a longer time to onset of action and can be given before the paralytics. Succinylcholine is commonly used for paralysis due to its short duration of action (<5 minutes), but should not be used in patients with burns, renal failure, Guillain–Barré syndrome, or end-stage renal disease because it can cause hyperkalemia. Nondepolarizing neuromuscular blocking agents have a longer duration of action, with the exception of rapacuronium, which may cause bronchospasm, hypotension, and tachycardia. Common induction agents and paralytics, their dosages, and time to onset of action are shown in **Table 5**.

Mechanical ventilation

Several modes of mechanical ventilation are now available with differing indications. The most commonly used modes are synchronized intermittent mandatory ventilation (SIMV) and continuous mandatory ventilation (CMV, also called assist control ventilation). These are volume-cycled modes and deliver a preset volume of gas to the patient. The pressure generated is directly proportional to the volume delivered, the airway resistance, and the lung and chest wall compliance. To avoid generation of dangerously high pressures, a pressure limit is set. When the inspiratory pressure reaches this level, a pressure relief ("pop-off") valve terminates inspiration and allows exhalation to begin.

Table 5. Agents used for intubation.

IV: intravenous; prn: *pro re nata* (as needed).

	Dosage (IV)	Onset of action	Duration
Induction agents			
Sodium thiopental	3–5 mg/kg hypotensive: 0.5–1 mg/kg	30–60 s	5–30 min
Etomidate	0.2–0.3 mg/kg hypotensive: 0.1–0.2 mg/kg	30–60 s	3–5 min
Ketamine	1–2 mg/kg	1–2 min	5–15 min
Propofol	0.25–2 mg/kg	30–60 s	3–10 min
Midazolam	1 mg, repeated prn	1–5 min	20–30 min
Lorazepam	1 mg, repeated prn	3–7 min	6–8 h
Paralytics			
Succinylcholine	1–1.5 mg/kg	1 min	3–5 min
Vecuronium	0.1 mg/kg	2.5–3 min	40 min
Cisatracurium	0.2 mg/kg	2–3 min	60 min
Rocuronium	0.3 mg/kg	1–2 min	30 min
Rapacuronium	1.5 mg/kg	1.5 min	<20 min

Time-cycled ventilation (pressure control ventilation [PCV]) is less commonly used, and generates an inspiratory flow for a preset time. An inspiratory pressure is set so the gas is delivered at a set pressure over a set time. When the airway pressure equals the inspiratory pressure flow ceases as there is no longer a pressure gradient. The tidal volume can fluctuate from breath to breath depending on the airway pressure. In flow-cycled ventilation (pressure support ventilation [PSV]), inspiration continues until a predetermined decrement in flow is achieved (typically 25% of initial flow). PSV can be used with SIMV to augment spontaneous breaths or, with CPAP, as a means of primary ventilation.

Modes of mechanical ventilation

Synchronized intermittent mandatory ventilation

SIMV is one of the most common ventilatory modes used. The physician prescribes the number of breaths to be delivered each minute, the tidal volume, the amount of PEEP, and often the PS. SIMV allows the patient to breathe spontaneously between breaths assisted by the ventilator. A patient who has no spontaneous respirations will have an RR equal to the machine rate. If the patient is taking spontaneous breaths, the ventilator will synchronize the machine breaths with inspiratory effort. If the patient is breathing at a faster rate than that set by the machine, those spontaneous breaths must be generated entirely by the patient. SIMV is particularly advantageous in a patient with asthma or COPD who is in respiratory distress with a high RR. These patients are at risk for dynamic hyperinflation, which results when the obstructive lung disease does not allow them to exhale the entire tidal volume before the next breath is delivered. If the ventilator delivers a full breath with each inspiratory effort in these patients, the patient may not be able to exhale each tidal volume leading to dynamic hyperinflation (auto-PEEP) and, potentially, barotrauma or hemodynamic instability.

Once a patient is placed on SIMV, the physician should evaluate the adequacy of the spontaneous breaths. A common mistake is to miss this step and set the PS at 10 cm H_2O and walk away. Many patients require a higher PS to ensure adequate tidal volumes during the spontaneous breaths, and low spontaneous tidal volumes can lead to increased work of breathing for a patient to achieve an adequate minute ventilation (MV). Therefore, the physician should simply observe the tidal volume during the spontaneous breath: if it is too low, the PS should be titrated until an adequate tidal volume is achieved. If given at a high enough level, PS can reduce the work of breathing a spontaneous breath to nearly zero; therefore, if the required PS is >20 cm H_2O, consideration can be given to switching to CMV to fully support each breath. In patients with COPD or asthma, care should be taken not to give such a large spontaneous tidal volume that dynamic hyperinflation develops.

Continuous mandatory ventilation

In CMV, or assist control ventilation, the ventilator delivers a preset volume every time the patient breathes, or it delivers a preset volume at a set rate, whichever is the higher frequency. CMV minimizes the work of breathing for the patient, and should, therefore, be used in the setting of myocardial ischemia or profound hypoxemia (where the work of breathing can increase oxygen consumption and worsen hypoxemia). One disadvantage to using CMV in patients who are tachypneic or have obstructive lung disease is that dynamic hyperinflation may occur if there is inadequate time to exhale the full tidal volume. Respiratory alkalosis may also develop in the tachypneic patient, and can result in myoclonus or seizures.

Pressure control ventilation

PCV differs from SIMV and CMV in that the physician sets an inspiratory pressure, not a tidal volume. During inspiration, a given pressure is imposed through the endotracheal tube (ETT), and the tidal volume delivered depends upon how much flow can be delivered prior to the airway pressure equilibrating with the inspiratory pressure. The tidal volume can vary from breath to breath; therefore, the minute volume is variable. PCV is typically used in patients with barotraumas (because the airway pressure can be limited) or acute respiratory distress syndrome (ARDS) or asthma (because airway pressures are intolerable on volume-cycled ventilation). Most patients must be heavily sedated or paralyzed to tolerate this mode of ventilation because they must passively accept ventilator breaths. During PCV for ARDS, the inspiratory to expiratory (I:E) ratio is often reversed (inverse-ratio ventilation). The I:E ratio is normally set at 1:2, allowing more time for exhalation, as is physiologic. But during PCV, increasing the length of inspiration can increase the amount of tidal volume delivered and improve gas exchange. Inverse ratio ventilation can use ratios of 1.5:1, 1.2:1, or 1:1, but cannot be used in obstructive lung disease such as asthma, because dynamic hyperinflation will result from the reduced time for exhalation.

Continuous positive airway pressure

CPAP is not a true form of mechanical ventilation, but provides a supply of fresh gas at a constant, specified pressure. It is most commonly used in weaning trials or in patients without respiratory failure who only require airway protection.

Pressure support ventilation

PSV is a patient-triggered mode of ventilation in which a preset pressure is maintained throughout inspiration. When inspiratory flow falls below a certain level, inspiration is terminated. PSV is commonly used in patients who require minimal support, or to assist the spontaneous breaths during SIMV or CPAP. If sufficient PS is used, patients can be fully supported and do very little work in order to breath. PS can initially be set at 10 cm H_2O and titrated according to the patient's spontaneous tidal volumes. The inspiratory flow rate (the rate at which the ventilator delivers each breath to the patient) is not usually prescribed by the physician, but set by the respiratory therapist, typically to 60 L/min, although it can be increased to 120 L/min. The physician should be aware that some patients require a higher flow rate than others. If a patient looks "air hungry" (is gasping or using accessory muscles during a machine-delivered breath) they may need a higher rate, and the inspiratory flow should be titrated to see if the patient could be made more comfortable. However, the higher flow rates will increase peak airway pressures, which could be limiting.

Airway pressure release ventilation

Airway pressure release ventilation is used in patients who are breathing spontaneously and are using CPAP. At the end of each ventilator cycle, the lungs are allowed to briefly deflate to ambient pressure and are then rapidly reinflated to the baseline (CPAP) pressure with the next breath. The perceived advantage of this technique is that lung expansion during exhalation is maintained with CPAP, but the brief interruption of this pressure at the end of exhalation allows for further CO_2 elimination, as well as enhanced venous return.

High frequency/jet ventilation

This mode of ventilation is used in neonates during intratracheal or intrabronchial surgery, and occasionally in patients with bronchopleural fistulas. This mode uses very small tidal volumes (50–150 mL) with very rapid rates (60–300 breaths/min).

Mechanical ventilation parameters

Once a mode of mechanical ventilation has been chosen, the physician must decide upon an RR, tidal volume, PEEP, oxygen concentration, and, occasionally, PS.

Minute ventilation

The normal MV for an adult at rest is approximately 5–6 L/min (MV = tidal volume × RR). When intubating a patient for the sole reason of decreased level of consciousness, the normal MV may be adequate to maintain gas exchange; however, in a profoundly ill patient, the MV requirements are typically much higher, and can approach 20 L/min.

Tidal volume

Traditionally, tidal volumes are set at 10–12 mL/kg/min; however, there has been a shift toward using lower tidal volume ventilation (4–8 mL/kg ideal body weight [IBW]/min) in patients with ALI as this has been proven to reduce mortality. Some physicians are using low tidal volume ventilation for all patients, even those who do not have ALI. Given the increasing evidence for barotrauma as a cause of morbidity and mortality, tidal volume should be limited in most patients, and should be initiated at 8 mL/kg/min.

Figure 1. Waveforms during dynamic hyperinflation. On the left side of the figure, volume and flow are shown during conventional volume-cycled ventilation with a square wave flow profile and no airflow obstruction. (Inspiratory flow is above the dashed, horizontal line.) On the right side of the figure, volume and flow are shown when significant expiratory obstruction and intrinsic positive end-expiratory pressure (PEEP) are present. Note the lower peak expiratory flow, the prolongation of expiration, and the presence of persistent expiratory flow at the onset of the subsequent breath. This persistent end-expiratory flow indicates the presence of intrinsic PEEP, shown on the volume plot as a raised functional residual capacity (FRC). The dashed curve (a) represents the continued fall in lung volume toward static FRC, which would occur if the subsequent breath were not given (or came later).

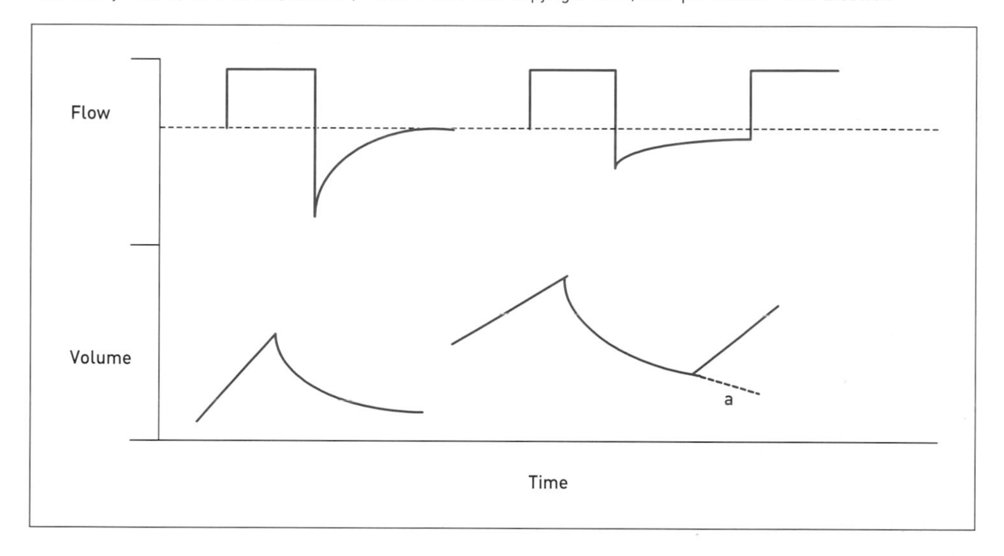

Respiratory rate

Once the tidal volume has been decided upon, the RR should be chosen to ensure adequate MV without causing dynamic hyperinflation. Patients with ARDS can typically tolerate an RR of up to 35 breaths/min because the stiff lungs recoil and exhale the tidal volume quickly, while in a patient with obstructive lung disease, a high RR can result in dynamic hyperinflation as another breath is delivered before the patient has time to exhale the entire tidal volume from the previous breath. This can be seen on the flow–volume curve (see **Figure 1**). When inspiration is triggered prior to the volume reaching zero, dynamic hyperinflation is present, and the RR and/or tidal volume should be decreased until this is corrected.

Dynamic hyperinflation has several negative consequences, including barotrauma and increased intrathoracic pressure. The latter can result in decreased venous return, decreased stroke volume, hypotension, and increased respiratory work (to trigger the ventilator, the patient normally has to generate a negative pressure; when dynamic hyperinflation is present, the patient must generate enough negative pressure to overcome the dynamic hyperinflation as well as generate the negative pressure). Serial arterial blood gas (ABG) analyses are required to ensure adequate gas exchange at the set minute volume.

Positive end-expiratory pressure

PEEP provides a continuous airway pressure above atmospheric pressure, preventing collapse of alveoli and small airways at end-expiration. By recruiting alveoli in this way, PEEP improves functional residual capacity and oxygenation.

PEEP is most commonly initiated at 5 cm H_2O. It can be titrated to 25 cm H_2O until adequate oxygenation is achieved, but the level of PEEP directly increases airway pressure, so high levels of PEEP can result in barotrauma or hypotension due to reduced venous return. When initially intubated, patients are typically placed on high oxygen concentration and weaned down to 50% as quickly as possible to prevent oxygen toxicity.

Monitoring during mechanical ventilation

Pulse oximetry

Pulse oximetry should be performed on all patients who are mechanically ventilated. However, caution should be exercised in patients who have CO poisoning or have experienced smoke inhalation, since the presence of carboxyhemoglobin falsely elevates the pulse oximetry because this technique cannot distinguish between oxyhemoglobin and carboxyhemoglobin. In this case, the partial pressure of O_2 (pO_2) as measured by an arterial blood gas should be monitored.

Arterial blood gas analysis

ABGs should be analyzed after any ventilator change that affects MV. ABGs do not have to be performed if fraction of inspired O_2 (FiO_2) is being titrated down, as long as the pulse oximetry is stable and correlates with the pO_2. In cases where FiO_2 is being persistently increased for hypoxemia, the ABG should be monitored to ensure adequate oxygenation.

Airway pressures

Airway pressures, including both peak airway pressure and plateau pressure, should be monitored closely. Peak airway pressure is the highest pressure reached during inspiration and is a function of both airway resistance and lung compliance. The plateau pressure is measured after an inspiratory pause (typically 0.5 seconds) at the end of inhalation, and is a function of the elastic recoil of the lung. The plateau pressure is a more reliable indicator of barotrauma and should be monitored regularly in the ventilated patient. Plateau pressures should be maintained at <30 cm H_2O, and this can be accomplished by reducing the tidal volume, reducing the PEEP (PEEP results in a 1:1 increase in plateau pressure), or correcting the underlying disease process. Assessment should be made for any correctable condition, as discussed below.

Troubleshooting ventilator problems

Several problems are frequently encountered during mechanical ventilation, the most common being elevated airway pressures, reduced tidal volumes, hypoxemia, and hypotension.

Elevated airway pressure

When treating a patient with elevated airway pressure, the physician should always evaluate both the peak inspiratory pressure and the plateau pressure. The difference between the peak

Figure 2. Algorithm for management of elevated airway pressures.

BS: breath sounds; CHF: congestive heart failure; ETT: endotracheal tube; nebs: nebulizers.

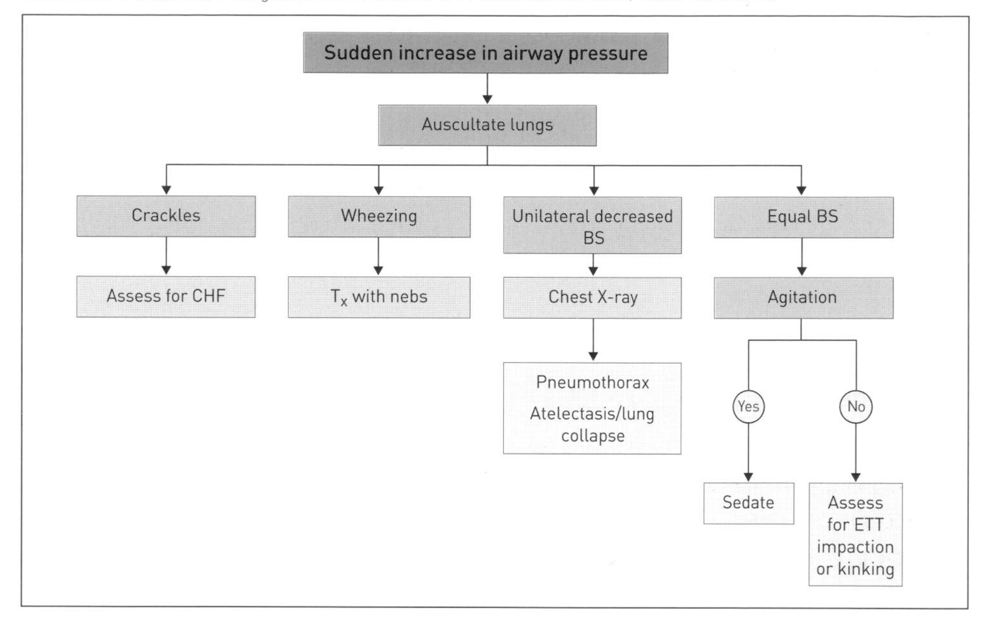

inspiratory and plateau pressures is the pressure that is required to overcome the resistance of the airways. If the peak pressure is significantly higher than the plateau pressure, then airway resistance is present, usually from bronchospasm, secretions, or kinking of the ETT. If the peak and plateau pressures are similar, or are rising in parallel, the patient is most likely experiencing reduced lung compliance, such as is seen in ARDS, CHF, pneumothorax, or right or left mainstem bronchus intubation. Elevated airway pressures can be seen from the start of intubation in patients with asthma, ARDS, CHF, or morbid obesity, but a rise in airway pressure should prompt a search for either a reversible cause or worsening of the underlying condition. Sudden increases in airway pressures can be caused by patient agitation, coughing, bronchospasm, mucous plugging, atelectasis, lung collapse, ETT occlusion, advancement of ETT into the right mainstem bronchus, or pneumothorax (see **Figure 2**).

Reduced tidal volume

A sudden decrease in tidal volume delivered during PCV usually indicates that there is elevated airway pressure, and that the set inspiratory pressure is being achieved with less tidal volume. Small tidal volumes during SIMV or CMV can occur with bronchospasm, increased secretions, decreased compliance, pneumothorax, dynamic hyperinflation, or an inappropriate I:E ratio. In the presence of a chest tube with a large air leak, the exhaled tidal volume may be low, as the ventilator does not monitor the leaking air.

Hypoxemia

Reduced oxygenation in a ventilated patient may be a ventilator-related problem, secondary to worsening of the underlying condition, or could represent a new complication (see **Table 6**). Any change in the patient's oxygenation should be evaluated promptly for a reversible cause.

Table 6. Causes of hypoxemia in ventilated patients.

ARDS: acute respiratory distress syndrome; CHF: congestive heart failure; COPD: chronic obstructive pulmonary disease; ETT: endotracheal tube.

Worsening of underlying disease	Ventilator problem	New complication
Pneumonia	Ventilator malfunction	Bronchospasm
ARDS	Incorrect settings	Atelectasis/lung collapse
COPD/asthma	Occluded ETT	Mucous plugs/secretions
CHF	ETT suctioning	Pneumothorax
		Pneumonia
		Pulmonary embolism
		Pulmonary edema
		Patient agitation

Table 7. Causes of hypotension in ventilated patients.

PEEP: positive end-expiratory pressure.

Ventilator related	Nonventilator related
Reduced venous return to heart	Left ventricular dysfunction
PEEP	Pericardial tamponade
Increased intrathoracic pressure (auto-PEEP)	Pulmonary embolism
Pneumothorax	Sepsis
	Volume depletion
	Medication related (sedatives/paralytics)

Hypotension

Hypotension is common in a critically ill, ventilated patient; however, if it is a new symptom, it should be evaluated. Most often, hypotension is not related to the ventilator but is related to other conditions, eg, septic shock, cardiogenic shock, hypovolemia, and, occasionally, anaphylaxis due to medication reaction. However, ventilator complications can lead to hypotension, and should be investigated, as they are readily reversible (see **Table 7**).

Weaning from mechanical ventilation

Patients should be evaluated daily to determine whether or not they are appropriate candidates for weaning. To be suitable for weaning, a patient should have an improvement or resolution of their underlying process, be awake and alert, off sedatives, and have no evidence of sepsis, hemodynamic instability, or acid–base imbalance. In addition, the ETT cuff should be deflated to assess for an air leak around the ETT; if no leak is audible, laryngeal edema may be present.

The rapid shallow breathing index (RSBI: RR/tidal volume) is the best marker for readiness to wean. The patient is placed on a pressure support of 0 cm H_2O with a PEEP of 5 cm H_2O and no set RR. After 1 minute, the RSBI is calculated. An RSBI of <100 indicates that weaning should be successful. Other weaning parameters are listed in **Table 8**. The three main weaning methods are T-piece trials, PS weaning, and SIMV weaning.

Table 8. Indications for a weaning trial.

Indications
Underlying condition improved
Patient is awake, alert, and cooperative
Gag reflex is intact
Rapid shallow breathing index <100 breaths/min
Respiratory rate <30 breaths/min
Minute ventilation <10 L/min
Negative inspiratory force <–20 cm H_2O

T-piece trials

T-piece trials consist of attaching the ETT to a T-piece (tubing with flow-by oxygen), when the indications for a weaning trial are met. If the patient tolerates this comfortably for 30 minutes with stable RR and stable heart rate, they can be extubated, although some physicians use a 2-hour trial. The patient must be closely monitored during this trial as he/she will be off the ventilator, and there will thus be no alarm to indicate low tidal volume or high RR.

Pressure support weaning

This is a modified version of the T-piece trial in which the patient is kept on the ventilator with a set RR of 0 breaths/min, pressure support of 5–10 cm H_2O, and a PEEP of 5 cm H_2O. If the patient shows a positive response for as little as 30 minutes, they can be extubated, although some physicians prefer to wait 2 hours.

SIMV weaning trials

SIMV weaning consists of decreasing the number of supported breaths by 1–2 breaths/min every 30 minutes for as long as the patient can tolerate. If they are stable at 0 breaths/min, they can then be extubated. SIMV weaning may result in more days on the ventilator than the weaning trials above and should not be the primary method of weaning.

Weaning failure

Signs of weaning failure include tachycardia, tachypnea, decreased tidal volumes, abdominal paradox (inward abdominal motion during inspiration), or patient distress. If the patient fails a weaning trial, they should be placed back on the ventilator and fully supported until the following day when another weaning trial may be attempted. A failed weaning trial should prompt a search for an underlying, unresolved problem that may be limiting the ability to extubate the patient.

Special situations

Two of the more difficult, but common, disease processes treated in the intensive care unit are ARDS and asthma. Management of patients with these conditions can be complicated.

ARDS

ARDS is defined by the acute onset of hypoxemic respiratory failure with bilateral infiltrates on chest X-ray, a pulmonary artery wedge pressure of <18 cm H_2O (or no clinical evidence of

Table 9. Risk factors for acute lung injury and acute respiratory distress syndrome.

Pulmonary causes	Nonpulmonary causes
Pneumonia	Sepsis
Aspiration	Systemic inflammatory response syndrome
Near-drowning	Shock
	Trauma
	Multiple blood transfusions
	Pancreatitis
	Burns
	Coronary artery bypass grafting
	Disseminated intravascular coagulation

left atrial hypertension), and a pO_2 in arterial blood (PaO_2)/FiO_2 ratio of <200. ALI is present when the above findings are present in the setting of a PaO_2/FiO_2 ratio of <300.

ALI and ARDS can develop in association with several conditions (see **Table 9**), not all of which directly involve the pulmonary system. The most common condition associated with ARDS is sepsis, with up to 40% of septic patients developing ARDS. Multiple risk factors increase the risk for ARDS synergistically.

Ventilator treatments for ARDS

Historically, treatment of ARDS has consisted of respiratory support and prompt resolution of the underlying or predisposing factor. Since sepsis is the most common cause of ARDS, a search for an undiagnosed infection should be undertaken if no clear etiology is present.

The primary mechanism of support is mechanical ventilation. Traditionally, tidal volumes used during mechanical ventilation were in the range of 12–15 mL/kg. ALI, which is similar to ARDS, has been observed in animals mechanically ventilated with large tidal volumes [5]. Ventilation with high airway pressures due to large tidal volumes has been shown to cause increased vascular permeability, acute inflammation, alveolar hemorrhage, and radiographic infiltrates. In patients with ALI or ARDS, the large tidal volumes are shunted to the unaffected areas of the lung because they provide the least resistance; this causes overdistention and damage to those previously unaffected segments.

The ARDSnet trial [6] showed that a "lung protective mechanism" of mechanical ventilation could improve survival. The goal of this approach is to provide adequate oxygenation while avoiding further trauma to the lung, which could worsen the existing injury. The ARDSnet trial was designed to assess whether lower tidal volumes and hence lower airway pressures would result in a clinical benefit in ARDS. This trial compared traditional ventilation (an initial tidal volume of 12 mL/kg IBW; IBW = 50 + 2.3[height in inches – 60] for males and 45.5 + 2.3[height in inches – 60] for females) with a lower tidal volume ventilation that started at 6 mL/kg IBW. In each group, the tidal volume was decreased in increments of 1 mL/kg IBW to maintain the plateau pressure below 50 cm H_2O for the traditional ventilation group and below 30 cm H_2O for the lower tidal volume group. The minimum tidal volume was 4 mL/kg IBW. PEEP and O_2 pressure were based on a sliding scale (see **Table 10**).

Table 10. Oxygen and positive end-expiratory pressure (PEEP) titration in the ARDSnet trial (the goal was a partial pressure of O_2 in arterial blood [PaO_2] of 55–80 mm Hg).

FiO_2: fraction of inspired oxygen.

FiO_2	PEEP (cm H_2O)	FiO_2	PEEP (cm H_2O)
0.3	5	0.7	14
0.4	5	0.8	14
0.4	8	0.9	14
0.5	8	0.9	16
0.5	10	0.9	18
0.6	10	1.0	20
0.7	10	1.0	22
0.7	12	1.0	24

The mortality rate was 39.8% in the group treated with traditional tidal volumes and 31.0% in the low tidal volume group (P=0.007); therefore, physicians should attempt to ventilate all patients with ARDS with low tidal volumes.

Because ARDS is a process that results in decreased lung compliance, patients can generally tolerate high RRs without the risk of dynamic hyperinflation, which is seen in obstructive diseases such as asthma or COPD. The ARDSnet trial used a maximum RR of 35 breaths/min. Despite this high rate, the low tidal volumes used to maintain plateau pressures below 30 cm H_2O resulted in respiratory acidosis in many patients, a result termed "permissive hypercapnia". When the arterial pH fell below 7.30 with a RR of 35 breaths/min, an infusion of sodium bicarbonate was started.

Low tidal volume ventilation clearly has an impact on the acid–base status of the patient, often resulting in significant acidosis in patients with renal failure who are unable to excrete their acid load. A patient on hemodialysis or continuous renal replacement therapy usually requires a higher concentration bicarbonate bath, as increasing the MV to improve acid–base control is often not an option. In some patients with severe ARDS, large infusions of bicarbonate may not improve acidosis. As hydrogen combines with bicarbonate, CO_2 is produced; the severely injured lungs may not be able to expel this adequately, resulting in worsening respiratory acidosis despite very high bicarbonate levels. Tris-hydroxymethyl aminomethane (THAM) is an alternative to bicarbonate; it is a buffer that accepts one proton per molecule, generating bicarbonate but not CO_2. THAM has been shown to control arterial pH without increasing CO_2 in the setting of refractory respiratory acidosis. THAM is excreted by the kidneys, so it is not recommended in patients with renal failure.

Nonventilator treatments for ARDS

Prone positioning has been advocated as a means to ventilate the posterior lung regions that are often atelectatic and flooded in ARDS. Once the patient is prone, these previously dependent lung regions open, as the anterior lung regions become dependent. Several personnel are required to safely move a patient into the prone position to ensure chest tubes, IV lines, and the ETT are not dislodged. Patients should be rotated every 12–18 hours. While prone positioning has been shown to improve gas exchange and oxygenation, it has not been shown to improve outcome.

The inflammatory response seen in ALI/ARDS has led to the evaluation of many anti-inflammatory agents as possible treatments. High doses of glucocorticoids have failed to prevent ARDS in high-risk patients and shown no benefit when given early in the course of the disease. However, they may show benefit in the late stages of ARDS, which are characterized by persistent inflammation and fibroproliferation.

Prostaglandin E_1, ketoconazole (an inhibitor of thromboxane and leukotriene synthesis), ibuprofen, and procysteine/*N*-acetylcysteine have all been evaluated and similarly found to have no benefit. Furthermore, treatment of sepsis prior to or early in the development of ALI/ARDS with an antiendotoxin monoclonal antibody, anti-tumor necrosis factor-α, or anti-interleukin (IL)-1, has also failed to show any benefit. Despite these discouraging results, studies using IL-10 and recombinant human platelet activating factor are currently in development.

Asthma

Asthma is very common, with 13 million people in the USA currently diagnosed with this disease. Severe asthma can occur in response to air pollutants, respiratory tract infections, exposure to allergens, or noncompliance with medication. Airway changes in severe asthma include bronchial smooth muscle contraction, bronchial inflammation with mucosal edema, and mucous plugging. These abnormalities lead to expiratory airflow obstruction. Severe obstruction can lead to dynamic hyperinflation, even in a nonventilated patient, as the tachypneic patient is not able to exhale their breaths by the next inspiration. This increases the work of breathing, and can result in respiratory muscle fatigue, which is the most common reason for respiratory failure in severe asthma.

Nonventilator treatments for asthma

Treatment of severe asthma includes β_2-agonist therapy, typically with albuterol nebulizers: 2.5–5 mg of albuterol should be given by nebulizer every 20 minutes for three doses, followed by 2.5–10 mg every 1–4 hours, depending on persistence of symptoms. Continuous nebulization with 10–15 mg/h is commonly used to treat severe asthma, and can be continued until asthma improves or side effects develop. Both intermittent and continuous modes have similar efficacy. Use of a metered dose inhaler (MDI) with a spacer can result in adequate delivery of albuterol if used correctly; however, nebulizers should be used in severe asthma as they require less cooperation from the potentially agitated patient.

Ipratropium is recommended for severe asthma in doses of 0.5 mg by nebulizer every 30 minutes for three doses, then every 2–4 hours as needed. This should be used in addition to albuterol, as ipratropium produces less bronchodilation. The nebulized dose can be combined with albuterol.

Subcutaneous terbutaline and epinephrine are occasionally used for severe asthma, although there has been no documented benefit from this therapy.

Corticosteroids are an important component of asthma treatment given the inflammatory nature of the disease. Intravenous methylprednisolone is recommended in doses of 120–240 mg/day in divided doses for 48 hours, followed by tapering based on the patient's condition. Improvement may be seen in as little as 1–2 hours.

Table 11. Pharmacological therapy for severe asthma.

IV: intravenous; nebs: nebulizers; prn: *pro re nata* (as needed).

Standard	Refractory asthma
Albuterol nebs 2.5–5 mg every 20 min × 3, then 2.5–10 mg every 1–4 h	Magnesium sulfate 2 g IV, then prn symptoms
Ipratropium nebs 0.5 mg every 30 min × 3, then every 2–4 h	Aminophylline bolus: 5 mg/kg (if no previous theophylline use) or: 0.5 mg/kg for each 1 µg/mL that theophylline level is <10 mg/mL (chronic users)
Methylprednisolone 60 mg IV every 6 h	Aminophylline drip: 0.6 µg/kg (goal level 6–12 mg/mL)

Theophylline acts as a bronchodilator, but has many side effects. Theophylline should not be used routinely in asthma as it has shown little benefit when added to albuterol [7]. Theophylline should be used in patients who are already using it on an outpatient basis, or in patients with severe disease refractory to other therapy.

Magnesium sulfate acts as a bronchodilator, and has shown benefit when given in a dose of 2 g IV to patients in the emergency department who have an initial forced expiratory volume in 1 second (FEV_1) of <30% of the predicted FEV_1 [8]. Magnesium sulfate can be used in patients who are not responding to the above therapy and have a life-threatening disease. In the nonventilated patient, the initial dose should be 2 g, and further doses require careful attention to side effects and serial magnesium levels. In patients with renal failure, inability to excrete magnesium via the kidneys will limit dosing. Pharmacological treatment for asthma is outlined in **Table 11**.

Heliox, a mixture of helium and oxygen that is available in mixtures of 60:40, 70:30, and 80:20, can be used to reduce airflow obstruction. Helium is less dense than air and decreases large airway resistance. If used, the 60:40 concentration should be initially tried, with careful monitoring of oxygenation.

Mechanical ventilation for asthma

Intubation and mechanical ventilation should be performed in asthmatic patients who develop mental status changes, cyanosis, or worsening respiratory acidosis despite therapy. Once a patient is intubated, he/she should be sedated with a benzodiazepine as well as an opioid to reduce the work of breathing and reduce tachypnea. The initial mode of mechanical ventilation should be SIMV, since ACV may lead to dynamic hyperinflation. The tidal volume should be 8–10 mL/kg IBW with an RR of 10–15 breaths/min, adjusted based on ABG analysis. The two problems most commonly encountered in the mechanically ventilated asthmatic are high peak airway pressures and dynamic hyperinflation.

High peak airway pressures

The high peak airway pressure typically reflects the severity of bronchoconstriction, and in severe asthma may limit the amount of tidal volume given. While peak airway pressures are higher than plateau pressures in asthma patients, it is the inspiratory plateau pressure that reflects the risk for barotrauma. A plateau pressure of >35 cm H_2O increases the risk for barotrauma, and should be avoided. Management of high airway pressures in an asthmatic patient should begin with adequate sedation, as agitation will increase airway pressure. If the patient is adequately sedated, nebulizers should be used frequently in addition to corticosteroids. The tidal volume should be minimized, while keeping the pH>7.20, and, as in ARDS, an infusion of sodium bicarbonate can be used to maintain the pH above this level.

A high inspiratory flow rate can increase peak pressures (but not plateau pressures). In contrast, a low inspiratory flow rate in volume-cycled ventilation can increase plateau pressures if it prolongs inspiration, resulting in shortened expiration and dynamic hyperinflation. If high airway pressures persist, paralysis should be considered, followed by aminophylline and, if elevated airway pressures continue, magnesium sulfate by IV infusion. If these measures do not work, pressure control ventilation can be utilized to bring the airway pressures under control, although the tidal volume may decrease. Inverse ratio ventilation (reversing the I:E ratio) should not be performed as the patient needs longer time for exhalation.

Dynamic hyperinflation occurs when an inspiratory breath is delivered to the patient who has not exhaled the entire tidal volume from the previous breath, and is discussed under the **Mechanical ventilation** section (see *page 7*). Resolution of dynamic hyperinflation requires either improving the underlying asthma or allowing more time for exhalation. Exhalation can be prolonged by decreasing the RR or the tidal volume. Both of these changes can result in worsening respiratory acidosis, and acid–base status should be followed with ABG analysis. If the inspiratory flow rate is <100 L/min, increasing the rate may reduce total inspiratory time and allow for longer exhalation, although increasing the flow rate above this level may hyperinflate areas of the lung that have less airway resistance, and could lead to barotrauma.

References

1. Mehta S, Jay GD, Woolard RH et al. Randomized, prospective trial of bilevel versus continuous positive airway pressure in acute pulmonary edema. *Crit Care Med* 1997;25:620–8.
2. International consensus conferences in critical care medicine: noninvasive positive ventilation in acute respiratory failure. *Am J Resp Crit Care Med* 2001;163:283–91.
3. Droner S, Merigian KS, Hedges JR et al. A comparison of blind nasotracheal and succinylcholine-assisted intubation in the poisoned patient. *Ann Emerg Med* 1987;16:650–2.
4. Macintyre NR. Principles of mechanical ventilation. In: Murray JF, Nadel JA, editors. *Textbook of Respiratory Medicine.* 3rd ed. Philadelphia, PA: Saunders, 2001:2471–86.
5. Parker JC, Hernandez LA, Peevy KJ. Mechanisms of ventilator induced lung injury. *Crit Care Med* 1993;21:131–43.
6. ARDS Network. Ventilation with lower tidal volumes as compared with traditional tidal volumes for acute lung injury and the acute respiratory distress syndrome. *N Engl J Med* 2000;1301–13.
7. Littenberg B. Aminophylline in severe, acute asthma. A meta-analysis. *JAMA* 1988;259:1678–84.
8. Silverman RA, Osborn H, Runge J et al. IV magnesium sulfate in the treatment of acute severe asthma: a multicenter randomized controlled trial. *Chest* 2002;122:489–97.

Part 2: Circulation

Matthew D Dollins

Anemia

Red blood cell transfusion

Anemia is very common in the critically ill patient and results in a very large number of blood transfusions. Traditionally, the 10/30 rule (a hemoglobin concentration of <10 g/dL or a hematocrit of <30%) has been the threshold for transfusion in hospitalized patients, but this was based more on decades of practice than clinical data. Concern over transmission of blood-borne pathogens and immunomodulatory effects of transfused red cells [1,2] has led to a reevaluation of this practice, and data are showing that most patients can tolerate lower hemoglobin and hematocrit levels.

There is currently no single "trigger point" for transfusion in all patients. The TRICC trial [3] demonstrated that reducing the transfusion threshold to a hemoglobin level of <7 g/dL is clinically as effective as using the higher threshold of <10 g/dL. This study randomized 838 critically ill patients to two groups: a liberal transfusion group, who were transfused at a hemoglobin level of <10 g/dL; and a restrictive transfusion group, who were only transfused at a hemoglobin level of <7 g/dL. Thirty-day mortality was similar in the two groups, but in-hospital mortality was lower in the restrictive group. Subgroup analysis of patients who were younger or less severely ill (age <55 or Acute Physiology and Chronic Health Evaluation [APACHE] II score of <20) showed a 50% decrease in mortality in the restrictive transfusion group. While this study suggests a lower transfusion threshold is as good as, and in some cases better than, a higher threshold, this practice does not appear to have been widely adopted. A recent observational study [4] of 4,892 patients found that 50% of patients admitted to intensive care units (ICUs) received transfusions, and that the mean pre-transfusion hemoglobin concentration was 8.6 g/dL.

The optimal transfusion threshold for patients with cardiovascular disease has also been debated. A large, combined retrospective and prospective study [5] found that patients admitted to ICUs with cardiac diagnoses (ischemic heart disease, arrhythmia, cardiac arrest, cardiac and vascular procedures) had a trend towards increased mortality when the hemoglobin concentrations were <9.5 g/dL. A retrospective study [6] of patients >65 years old with acute MI showed that transfusing patients with a hematocrit of <30% can reduce 30-day mortality. However, subgroup analysis [7] of the TRICC trial showed that in patients with cardiovascular disease there was no difference in mortality between those who were transfused at a hemoglobin threshold of <10 g/dL and those transfused at <7 g/dL.

No single level can currently be set that should trigger transfusion in all patients. Clinical assessment and careful monitoring of a patient's status must guide the physician in deciding when to transfuse. A lower threshold for transfusion would be appropriate for most patients, while

Table 1. Classification of shock.

AAA: abdominal aortic aneurysm.

Hypovolemic	Distributive	Cardiogenic	Extracardiac obstructive
Blood losses Internal hemorrhage: - spleen/liver laceration - aortic dissection - AAA rupture - pelvis/long-bone fracture - ruptured ectopic pregnancy External hemorrhage: - trauma - massive hematuria - gastrointestinal bleeding **Fluid losses** - diarrhea - vomiting - diabetic ketoacidosis - burns - adrenal crisis **Volume depletion** - debilitated patient - comatose/found down	Sepsis Anaphylaxis Neurogenic shock	Myocardial infarction Myocarditis Acute mitral regurgitation Rupture of interventricular septum Hypertrophic cardiomyopathy	Pericardial tamponade Massive pulmonary embolism Pulmonary hypertension

patients with cardiovascular disease (and likely cerebrovascular disease as well) should have their hematocrits maintained at a level of at least 30%.

Erythropoietin therapy

The two main factors resulting in anemia in the ICU are phlebotomy and inadequate red blood cell production. Critically ill patients exhibit reduced erythropoietin production and a reduced erythropoietin response [8], which is largely due to the suppression of erythropoietin gene expression and red blood cell production by inflammatory cytokines.

Recombinant human erythropoietin (rHuEPO) can reduce the need for transfusion in the critically ill patient, as was recently demonstrated in a randomized, controlled trial [9]. Either placebo or 40,000 units of rHuEPO was given subcutaneously per week, starting on ICU day 3, for a total of three doses (patients in the ICU on study day 21 received a fourth dose). Treatment with rHuEPO resulted in a 10% absolute reduction in the number of patients requiring red cell transfusions (60.4% for placebo vs. 50.5% for rHuEPO), and a 19% reduction in the total units transfused to the rHuEPO group. While reducing the number of transfusions required, rHuEPO did not change clinical outcomes (including mortality rate, rate of organ failure, and length of stay in the ICU), and has yet to gain widespread recommendation for routine use. When treating hemodynamically unstable patients with rHuEPO, one might consider intravenous administration since the patients' ability to absorb subcutaneous medications could be impaired.

Table 2. Hemodynamic changes in shock.

BP: blood pressure; SVR: systemic vascular resistance.

Classification	BP	Cardiac output	Wedge pressure	SVR
Cardiogenic shock	↓↓	↓↓	↑↑	↑
Cardiogenic shock due to right ventricular infarction	↓↓	↓↓	Normal/↓	↑
Extracardiac obstructive shock	↓↓	↓	↑↑	↑
Pericardial tamponade	↓↓	↓	↑	↑
Massive pulmonary embolism	↓↓	↓	Normal	↑
Hypovolemic shock	↓↓	↓	↓	↑↑
Septic shock	↓↓	↑	Normal/↓	↓↓

Table 3. Fluids used for resuscitation.

Fluid	Sodium (mEq/L)	Chloride (mEq/L)	Potassium (mEq/L)	Osmolarity (mOsm/L)	Oncotic pressure (mm Hg)	Lactate (mEq/L)	Maximum dose (mL/kg/day)	Cost (US$/L)
Sodium chloride (0.9%)	154	154	0	308	0	0	None	1.26
Ringer's lactate	130	109	4	275	0	28	None	1.44
Sodium chloride (3%)	513	513	0	1025	0	0	Limited by serum Na^+	1.28
Albumin (5%)	130–160	130–160	0	310	20	0	None	100
Hetastarch (6%)	154	154	0	310	30	0	20	27.30
Dextran 70 + NaCl 0.9%	154	154	0	310	60	0	20	35.08
Urea-gelatin	145	145	5.1	391	26–30	0	20	–

Shock

Shock occurs when the circulatory system is unable to maintain adequate cellular perfusion, which results in an imbalance of oxygen delivery and consumption in the tissues. Shock is a clinically defined syndrome and is classified into four main groups (see **Table 1**): hypovolemic shock; distributive shock; cardiogenic shock; and extracardiac obstructive shock.

The unifying feature of all of these groups is hypotension leading to decreased cellular perfusion, with resulting cellular hypoxia/anoxia. Cellular hypoxia/anoxia can lead to end-organ failure, such as acute renal failure, hepatic failure, encephalopathy, gut ischemia, myocardial infarction (MI), and gangrene of the extremities.

Table 4. Potential disadvantages of colloids.

Albumin	Negative inotropic effect [11] Impaired salt and water excretion [12] Increased mortality [13]
Hetastarch	Acute renal failure in setting of sepsis [14] Increased serum amylase levels
Dextrans	Anaphylactic reaction due to histamine release [15]
Hypertonic saline	Hypernatremia

Clinical manifestations of shock

Many manifestations of shock are similar irrespective of the underlying cause. Hypotension is universal, and tachycardia, tachypnea, confusion, cool extremities, and metabolic acidosis are very common. **Table 2** shows the hemodynamic changes characteristic of each form of shock.

General principles for managing shock

Fluids

Most patients who are in shock require large volumes of intravenous fluids. Patients with hypovolemic shock have a large fluid deficit, those with septic shock have vasodilatation and venous pooling as well as transudation of large amounts of fluid into the extravascular space, and even some patients in cardiogenic shock may need fluids to maximize cardiac output. The types of fluids used are quite varied (see **Table 3**), and controversy exists as to which agent is best. Both crystalloids (electrolyte solutions) and colloids (high-molecular-weight solutions) are used to treat shock.

Crystalloids

Isotonic crystalloid solutions have traditionally been the preferred fluids for volume expansion. Normal saline (0.9%) and lactated Ringer's solution are both commonly used, although large volumes of lactated Ringer's solution should be avoided in the setting of renal failure as it can result in hyperkalemia. Large volumes should also be avoided in patients with hepatic failure because the damaged liver may not be able to convert lactate to bicarbonate. One advantage of isotonic crystalloids is that they replace the interstitial fluid deficits seen after hypovolemic shock: 75% of the volume infused enters the interstitial space, while 25% remains intravascular. However, large volumes of these fluids are required, leading to peripheral edema, which may impair wound healing. This has led to the study of hypertonic crystalloid and colloid solutions, which stay within the intravascular space to a greater degree, and thus require less total volume for a similar degree of resuscitation.

Hypertonic crystalloid solutions include 3%, 5%, and 7.5% sodium chloride, and are considered plasma expanders because they act to increase the circulatory volume via movement of intracellular and interstitial water into the intravascular space. The primary disadvantage of these agents is the risk of hypernatremia, and their safety depends partially on how much water can be shifted from the intracellular to the extracellular space (to compensate for the increased extracellular osmolality) without resulting in cellular damage.

Table 5. Vasopressor characteristics.

[a]Dopamine may cause intestinal ischemia at 2 μg/kg/min; low-dose dopamine is considered 1–3 μg/kg/min.

Agent	Dose	Cardiac effects	Peripheral effects
Dopamine	1–3 μg/kg/min[a] 3–5 μg/kg/min 5–20 μg/kg/min	+ + ++	0/+ + ++
Norepinephrine	2–30 μg/min	+	+++
Phenylephrine	20–200 μg/min	0	+++
Epinephrine	1–20 μg/min	+++	+++
Dobutamine	2–20 μg/kg/min	+++	0 (vasoconstriction) ++ (vasodilation)
Vasopressin	0.04 U/min	Unknown in shock	++

Colloids

Colloids are also plasma expanders, as they are composed of macromolecules, and are retained in the intravascular space to a much greater extent than isotonic crystalloids. Albumin increases intravascular oncotic pressure, and may protect the lungs and other organs from edema. Dextran is a colloid agent prepared from glucose polymers, and is available as dextran 40 and dextran 70. Hydroxyethyl starch (HES, or hetastarch) is available in different preparations (HES 200 or HES 450). HES is a natural starch of highly branched glucose polymers, similar in structure to glycogen. Its volume expansion properties are almost identical to those of albumin. Pentastarch has a higher colloid oncotic pressure than HES or albumin, thus producing more intravascular volume expansion than these two agents. Recent evidence shows that the starches may be able to reduce capillary leak following ischemia or trauma, thereby decreasing edema formation [10]. Gelatins are polypeptides from bovine raw material, and are poorly retained in the intravascular space. Their duration of effect is approximately 2 hours. Gelatins are not available in the USA at this time. Newer solutions consisting of hypertonic saline to which colloids have been added include NaCl 7.5% with dextran 70, NaCl 7.2% with dextran 60, and NaCl 7.5% with hetastarch.

Crystalloids vs. colloids for resuscitation

There has been much debate as to which type of fluid is best to use for resuscitation of shock. Colloids offer the theoretical advantage of expanding the intravascular space with less volume, and have been shown to increase blood pressure more rapidly than crystalloids: 1 L of dextran 70 increases intravascular volume by 800 mL; 1 L of HES by 750 mL; 1 L of 5% albumin by 500 mL; and 1 L of saline by 180 mL. However, in the setting of sepsis, where there is often significant capillary leak, the benefit from colloids may be lost. Colloids also have several potential side effects that make them less attractive (see **Table 4**), and most studies have not found a benefit for colloids over crystalloids.

Given the available data and potential risks of colloid solutions, crystalloids remain the cornerstone of volume resuscitation, although patients with profound volume deficits may benefit from colloid solutions in addition to crystalloids to accelerate restoration of circulating volume.

Vasopressors

Despite adequate fluid resuscitation, many patients remain in shock and require vasopressor agents (see **Table 5**). Dopamine is widely used, and the Society of Critical Care Medicine guidelines recommend dopamine as the agent of first choice [16]. However, it can cause tachycardia and arrhythmias, which may limit its use. Norepinephrine is as effective in raising blood pressure as dopamine, but has fewer cardiac effects; it does not raise cardiac output as much as dopamine, and causes less tachycardia. Phenylephrine has purely α-adrenergic blocking effects, and is associated with less risk of tachyarrhythmia. Epinephrine can be used for refractory hypotension, but has been shown to cause a rise in serum lactate levels.

Dobutamine has been used in sepsis to improve oxygen delivery, but can potentiate hypotension due to β_2-mediated vasodilatation. Dobutamine is recommended for patients with a low cardiac index (<2.5 L/min/m^2) after volume resuscitation, but if profound hypotension is present (a systolic blood pressure [SBP] of <80 mm Hg) it should be used in conjunction with an agent with more peripheral vasoconstrictor effects, such as norepinephrine or phenylephrine. Vasopressin (also called antidiuretic hormone) causes vasoconstriction by activating V_1 receptors on vascular smooth muscle cells. However, experience with vasopressin in the setting of shock is limited. While one small study has shown vasopressin to improve blood pressure in septic shock [17], others have suggested it can cause a reduction in cardiac output [18].

Treatment of acidosis

Lactic acidosis due to tissue hypoperfusion is common in shock. Improvement of the effective circulating volume and restoring tissue oxygen balance will diminish the production of lactate, allowing improvement of acidosis. However, in cases of intractable shock, metabolic acidosis may persist despite aggressive therapy.

In animal models, acidosis has been shown to decrease cardiac contractility [19], and to reduce cardiac contractility in response to catecholamines. However, the effect of acidosis on human cardiac function in the clinical setting is less well documented. Decreased cardiac contractility in the setting of lactic acidosis may partially be due to hypoxemia, hypoperfusion, or sepsis, and establishing the direct effects of the low pH are difficult. Indeed, many patients treated with permissive hypercapnia/low tidal volume ventilation develop acidosis that is well tolerated with minimal change in cardiac output.

Treatment of acidosis with sodium bicarbonate has not been shown to be beneficial. In animal models of lactic acidosis, sodium bicarbonate failed to improve hemodynamics compared with normal saline [20,21], and human studies have shown no improvement in hemodynamics or catecholamine responsiveness [22,23]. Furthermore, bicarbonate infusion may in fact worsen intracellular acidosis: the carbon dioxide produced when bicarbonate reacts with acids can diffuse rapidly across the cell membrane, whereas bicarbonate cannot. Treatment of acidosis with bicarbonate has also been shown to increase hemoglobin's affinity for oxygen in healthy volunteers, resulting in reduced oxygen delivery.

Since there is no documented benefit, and the potential for adverse effects appears real, treatment of lactic acidosis should not include administration of sodium bicarbonate.

Table 6. Compensatory response to shock.

2,3-DPG: 2,3-diphosphoglycerate; RBC: red blood cell.

Maximize intravascular volume	Redistribution of fluid to intravascular space: – from interstitial compartments – from intracellular compartments Renal adaptations: – increased aldosterone – increased vasopressin
Maximize blood pressure	Increased sympathetic activity Increased catecholamines Increased angiotensin II production Increased vasopressin
Maximize cardiac output	Sympathetic stimulation: – tachycardia – increased contractility
Maximize oxygen delivery	Metabolic acidosis Increased RBC 2,3 DPG Decreased tissue oxygen levels

Hypovolemic shock

Hypovolemic shock is defined as a reduction in effective circulating blood volume, which leads to an oxygen deficit in the tissues because oxygen supply is not able to meet oxygen demand. This imbalance in oxygen metabolism leads to cellular ischemia, and, if prolonged, cellular death. Hypovolemic shock occurs most commonly as a result of trauma and hemorrhage, but can also be seen in other conditions (see **Table 1**).

Pathogenesis

Loss of circulating volume is the primary stimulus for the manifestation of hypovolemic shock. Once 10% of circulating volume has been lost, compensatory mechanisms are activated to maintain cardiac output despite the decreased ventricular filling pressures and stroke volume (see **Table 6**). Sympathetic discharge and adrenal catecholamine release lead to tachycardia and arterial vasoconstriction and venoconstriction. As volume loss increases, the increase in heart rate is not able to overcome the loss of stroke volume, and cardiac output declines, which is initially detected as orthostatic hypotension and a fall in pulse pressure. Once the loss of volume exceeds approximately 40%, or 20%–25% if lost rapidly, hypotension and shock ensue.

Clinical manifestations

Early in the course of hypovolemia or blood loss the patient may not be hypotensive, so attention should be paid to other signs of fluid loss such as tachycardia and tachypnea. Orthostatic hypotension is also a reliable sign, while dry mucosal membranes and decreased skin turgor are less reliable. If the patient is conscious, he/she may complain of thirst or diaphoresis. Once volume loss becomes profound, hypotension ensues, and the patient may become confused and develop oliguria and peripheral cyanosis as a result of diminished perfusion. Hypovolemic shock due to trauma or bleeding is usually apparent, but internal bleeding or other causes (as listed in **Table 1**) may not be as obvious. The smell of acetone on the patient's breath may indicate uncontrolled diabetes mellitus, while adrenocortical insufficiency can result in brown discoloration of the mucous membranes.

Figure 1. Spectrum of systemic inflammatory response syndrome (SIRS), sepsis, septic shock, and multiple organ dysfunction syndrome (MODS).

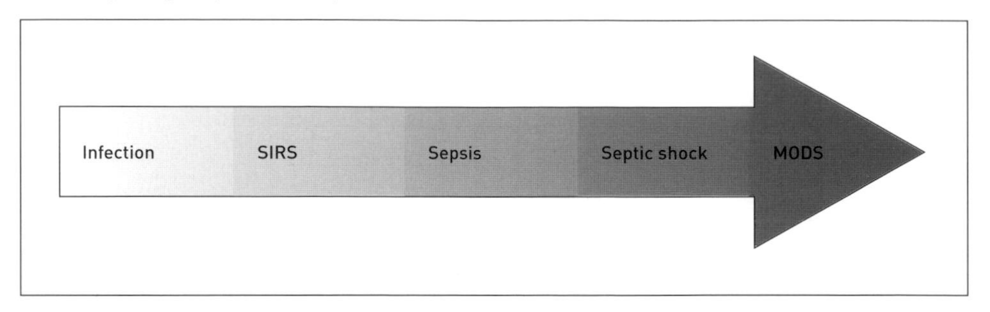

Acidosis often occurs due to hypoperfusion of tissues, which results in lactate production. Disseminated intravascular coagulation (DIC) can also occur during hypovolemic shock, resulting in microvascular thrombi formation, and may contribute to the multiple organ dysfunction syndrome (MODS) often seen following traumatic or hypovolemic shock.

Cellular ischemia in the gut may result in gastric ulcers, as well as disruption of the barrier function of the mucosa, which can result in translocation of bacteria from the bowel into the circulation. Hepatic ischemia can decrease the clearance of lactate and drugs, and centrilobular necrosis may result in elevated bilirubin and transaminase levels. The spleen contracts during hypovolemic shock, releasing red blood cells into the circulation. Myocardial ischemia can occur, particularly in elderly patients who may have atherosclerotic coronary artery disease. Renal failure is common.

Diagnosis

The initial evaluation of the patient in shock should include a determination of the cause. In most cases of hypovolemic shock, it is readily apparent that trauma or blood loss is the primary cause, but care must be taken not to overlook septic, cardiogenic, or anaphylactic shock. Initial resuscitation should begin during the evaluation. In the case of external blood loss, blood should be cross-matched while fluids are infused for resuscitation. Gastrointestinal bleeding can be evaluated and potentially treated with upper or lower endoscopy, or evaluated with angiography once the patient is stabilized. In the event of trauma, a chest X-ray should be performed to rule out tension pneumothorax or hemothorax. If abdominal trauma has occurred, peritoneal lavage can be performed to assess for hemorrhage, which is most commonly caused by splenic or hepatic lacerations.

If the patient is stabilized, computerized tomography or ultrasound can be used to look for and assess intra-abdominal hemorrhage and organ injury. Laboratory tests should include complete blood count; a chemistry panel including electrolytes, creatinine, glucose, and liver function tests; arterial blood gas; arterial lactate level; blood type and crossmatch; and urinalysis. In the event of trauma or bleeding, coagulation studies should include platelet count, prothrombin time, and partial thromboplastin time. If the cause of shock is not readily apparent, an electrocardiogram (ECG) should be performed to rule out MI.

Table 7. Definition of systemic inflammatory response syndrome (SIRS), sepsis, severe sepsis, septic shock, and multiple organ dysfunction syndrome (MODS).

WBC: white blood cell.

SIRS	Presence of two or more of the following: - temperature >38°C or <36°C - heart rate >90 beats/min - respiratory rate >20 breaths/min - WBC count >20,000 cells/mm^3, <4,000 cells/mm^3 - >10% immature neutrophils
Sepsis	SIRS in the presence of suspected or documented infection
Severe sepsis	Sepsis with hypotension, hypoperfusion, or organ dysfunction
Septic shock	Sepsis with hypotension unresponsive to volume resuscitation, and evidence of hypoperfusion or organ dysfunction
MODS	Dysfunction of more than one organ

Management

Resuscitation of the patient in shock should begin immediately, and should not be delayed while diagnostic procedures are undertaken. Fluid resuscitation should begin once large-bore intravenous catheters are placed. The primary goal in the treatment of hypovolemic shock is to return circulating volume to normal and, as a result, improve tissue perfusion, substrate delivery, and oxygen balance. Fluid resuscitation is the initial therapy in hypovolemic shock, as this helps restore circulating volume and oxygen delivery.

The use of vasopressors in hypovolemic shock should be reserved for circumstances in which adequate fluids are not yet available, or for patients in whom adequate fluid infusion has not improved hypotension. In this setting, a pulmonary artery catheter can help guide therapy as persistent shock can be caused by either peripheral vasodilatation or myocardial dysfunction. A wedge pressure of 12–16 mm Hg is indicative of adequate volume expansion.

Animal studies have shown that vasopressin can reverse shock that is unresponsive to fluids and catecholamines, and can improve survival after cardiac arrest in hypovolemic shock [24]. However, only case reports of improvement in human hypovolemic shock are available.

Distributive shock

Distributive shock is characterized by a severe decrease in the systemic vascular resistance. Septic shock is the most common form of distributive shock, and is the only form that will be discussed here. Anaphylactic and neurogenic shock should be considered in the appropriate setting.

Septic shock

It is estimated that sepsis accounts for up to 10% of ICU admissions and that there are 750,000 episodes of sepsis each year in the USA, resulting in >200,000 deaths per annum [25].

Definition

Septic shock is part of a continuum that begins with an infection followed by the systemic inflammatory response syndrome (SIRS) (see **Figure 1**). SIRS, sepsis, severe sepsis, septic shock, and MODS are defined in **Table 7**.

Source of infection and microbiology

The infectious causes of sepsis include Gram-negative organisms (25%), Gram-positive organisms (25%), mixed Gram-positive and Gram-negative organisms (20%), fungi (3%), anaerobic organisms (2%), and organisms unknown (25%) [26]. The Gram-negative organisms most commonly associated with sepsis are *Escherichia coli* (25%), *Klebsiella* (20%), and *Pseudomonas aeruginosa* (15%). The Gram-positive organisms most commonly associated with sepsis are *Staphylococcus aureus* (35%), *Enterococcus* (20%), and coagulase-negative *Staphylococcus* (15%). The most common primary sites of infection in sepsis are the respiratory tract (50%), intra-abdominal area/pelvis (20%), urinary tract (10%), skin (5%), and intravascular catheters (5%) [26].

There has been a rise in the incidence of sepsis and septic shock over the last few decades. Factors that may be responsible include the increase in interventional procedures and the increasing number of immunocompromised patients either due to HIV/AIDS or because of cytotoxic or immunosuppressant therapy. Other risk factors for sepsis include malnutrition, alcoholism, malignancy, diabetes mellitus, advanced age, and chronic kidney disease.

Pathophysiology

Inflammatory system

The manifestations of sepsis are believed to result from an excessive inflammatory response to bacterial organisms. Both proinflammatory and anti-inflammatory cytokines are released in response to bacterial invasion, and these two systems are usually tightly controlled to destroy the infection while preventing damage to the host. Sepsis results from an imbalance between these two processes, with the proinflammatory component being overexpressed; however, studies in critically ill patients have shown that neutrophils demonstrate functional abnormalities that may impair host defense. Whether or not this neutrophil dysfunction leads to worsening of the sepsis syndrome is unknown.

Coagulation system

Sepsis is characterized by a prothrombotic and antifibrinolytic state. Protein C levels are decreased, and conversion of protein C to activated protein C, which inhibits thrombosis, is impaired. Levels of antithrombin III and of tissue factor pathway inhibitor, which inhibits the highly thrombogenic compound tissue factor, have also been found to be reduced in the setting of sepsis. These factors contribute to the widespread microvascular thrombosis that occurs during sepsis, leading to hypoperfusion in various tissues and subsequent MODS, which is seen in many patients with sepsis.

Clinical features

Systemic manifestations

Common clinical manifestations include changes in body temperature (fever or hypothermia), tachycardia, tachypnea, and leukocytosis or leukopenia. Hypoglycemia, hyperglycemia, and impaired electrolyte balance can also be seen. Patients with severe sepsis and septic shock have hypotension due to decreased effective circulating volume. The intravascular volume depletion is related to several factors, including decreased systemic vascular resistance (SVR), increased microvascular permeability, and increased insensible losses.

Cardiovascular manifestations

Findings from pulmonary artery catheterization show that once volume resuscitation has been achieved, most patients with septic shock exhibit hyperdynamic cardiovascular function with a normal or elevated cardiac output and decreased SVR. However, the heart may not be as hyperdynamic as expected considering the clinical setting. Sepsis can induce depression of myocardial function, characterized by elevated left ventricular end-diastolic volume and a decreased left ventricular systolic work index. This myocardial depression is thought to be due to release of a myocardial depressant substance, which has not yet been identified, although tumor necrosis factor (TNF)-α and interleukin (IL)-1 are leading candidates.

Pulmonary manifestations

Up to 40% of patients with sepsis have been reported to have ARDS, and tachypnea and hypoxemia are also common in this patient group. Many view ARDS as an initial manifestation of MODS and believe it represents diffuse endothelial injury resulting from the exaggerated inflammatory response.

Adrenocortical manifestations

Adrenal insufficiency is a common finding in septic shock, with a reported incidence of 25%–40%. The threshold for diagnosing adrenal insufficiency is a cortisol level of 25–30 μg/mL instead of the usual 18–20 μg/mL. The low-dose adrenocorticotrophic hormone (ACTH) stimulation test (1–2 μg) should be used for the diagnosis of adrenal insufficiency, as it represents physiologic stress levels of ACTH, in contrast to the standard ACTH stimulation test, which uses doses that are 100–200-fold higher than maximal stress levels of ACTH. In a fluid-resuscitated patient who is hypotensive and requiring vasopressors, a randomly assessed cortisol level of <25 μg/mL should be considered diagnostic of adrenal insufficiency.

Vascular manifestations

DIC is often seen in sepsis and is characterized by enhanced activation of coagulation, along with intravascular fibrin formation and deposition. The resulting microvascular thrombi can reduce blood flow to portions of organs, thus contributing to the onset of MODS. A reduction in circulating coagulation factors and platelets is often seen as these components are consumed in the production of microthrombi, and this can lead to bleeding episodes. Laboratory studies of DIC typically show thrombocytopenia, with an elevation of prothrombin time, activated partial thromboplastin time, and D-dimer levels.

Nervous system manifestations

Central nervous system alterations are often seen in patients with sepsis, and septic encephalopathy is the most common form of encephalopathy in the ICU. Confusion, disorientation, lethargy, agitation, obtundation, and coma are the most common clinical manifestations.

Critical illness polyneuropathy is a common occurrence in the setting of sepsis, and is often first recognized when the patient cannot be weaned from ventilatory support. This illness is characterized by hyporeflexia, distal weakness (as opposed to proximal weakness), and normal or slightly elevated creatine kinase levels. Recovery may take up to 6 months.

Renal manifestations

Renal dysfunction is found in 9%–40% of patients with sepsis; the mortality rate in these patients is >50%. The clinical manifestations vary from acute tubular necrosis to bilateral cortical necrosis. Hypotension is commonly seen in sepsis, and renal hypoperfusion plays a major role in the incidence of acute renal failure (ARF), as does the administration of nephrotoxic agents such as aminoglycosides to treat sepsis. Elevated cytokine levels may contribute to ARF by causing renal vasoconstriction.

MODS

As the standard of care for critically ill patients has improved, death from the initial disease process in sepsis has become less common, patients have lived longer, and the development of MODS has become more common. MODS is now the most common cause of death among patients with sepsis. The exact pathophysiologic mechanism leading to MODS has not been fully defined, but mitochondrial dysfunction, microvascular thrombi, hypoperfusion, ischemia–reperfusion injury, circulating inflammatory factors, diffuse endothelial cell injury, bacterial toxin translocation, and increased tissue nitric oxide levels are all potential contributors.

Management

The management of sepsis is primarily based on eradication of the infection and support of the patient's hemodynamics and organ systems.

Antibiotics

Identifying the source of sepsis should be one of the primary goals while treatment is being initiated. Antibiotic choice often depends on the suspected site of infection. Initial antibiotic therapy should include broad-spectrum coverage of Gram-positive organisms and double antibiotic coverage of Gram-negative organisms until a source can be identified. Once the source is identified, coverage can be targeted to the cultured organism or the clinical situation. If no organism is isolated, initial broad-spectrum antibiotics can be continued as long as the patient is improving. Immediate institution of antibiotic therapy is critical since there is a 10%–15% higher mortality rate in patients who are not given treatment promptly [27].

Hemodynamic support

Intravascular volume depletion, peripheral vasodilatation, and increased microvascular permeability all contribute to hypotension in patients with severe sepsis and septic shock, and aggressive volume resuscitation should be the primary initial therapy; delaying resuscitation will increase the risk of organ failure. The fluid requirements for resuscitation are large, and are often underestimated by the clinician. Up to 10 L of crystalloid are often required in the first 24 hours. Boluses of fluid should be given until blood pressure, heart rate, or evidence of end-organ perfusion – such as urine output – has improved. Crystalloids, such as normal saline, are the fluids of choice for volume resuscitation; albumin is not recommended, as discussed earlier.

Despite adequate fluid resuscitation, many patients remain hypotensive, and these patients require vasopressor agents. Dopamine and norepinephrine are the first choices, and other agents can be incorporated into the regimen if the patient remains hypotensive.

Treatment of the underlying condition will accelerate resolution of DIC. No specific therapy is recommended for DIC unless severe or life-threatening hemorrhage occurs, at which time replacement with platelets, fresh/frozen plasma, and possibly cryoprecipitate are indicated.

Activated protein C

The finding that protein C levels are reduced in sepsis and are associated with an increased risk of death led to the study of activated protein C (APC) in the treatment of sepsis. The PROWESS trial [28] was a large, randomized, double-blind, placebo-controlled, multicenter trial that evaluated the effects of recombinant human APC (drotrecogin alfa [activated]) in patients with severe sepsis. The criteria for severe sepsis were presence of a known or suspected infection, three or more signs of SIRS, and at least one organ dysfunction. Patients were treated with placebo (n=840) or a continuous infusion of drotrecogin alfa (activated) (n=850) for 96 hours. Patients treated with drotrecogin alfa (activated) had a 19.4% reduction in the relative risk of death, and an absolute risk reduction of 6.1%. PROWESS was the first randomized controlled trial to show a survival benefit of a therapeutic intervention in sepsis.

The US Food and Drug Administration has approved drotrecogin alfa (activated) for adult patients with severe sepsis and a high risk of death (an APACHE II score of ≥25). A study is in progress to assess the efficacy of drotrecogin alfa (activated) in patients with an APACHE II score of <25. Because drotrecogin alfa (activated) has anticoagulant properties, there is an increased risk of bleeding associated with its use, and the incidence of serious bleeding in the treated group in PROWESS was higher than in the controls (3.5% vs. 2.0%) despite stringent criteria to exclude those at risk for bleeding. Drotrecogin alfa (activated) should be considered for all patients at high risk for death from sepsis, with three SIRS criteria, and at least one organ dysfunction. Patients with conditions that were exclusion criteria in the PROWESS trial (including pregnancy, breast feeding, chronic kidney disease requiring dialysis, acute pancreatitis without a known source of infection, cirrhosis, and HIV infection with a $CD4^+$ T cell count of <50 cells/mm^3) should be evaluated carefully. Care should also be taken in patients who are at risk for bleeding. A recent safety assessment by Bernard et al. indicates that invasive procedures are associated with a substantial percentage of serious bleeding events, particularly those occurring at the start of drotrecogin alfa (activated) infusion [29]. Further risk factors for serious bleeding include severe thrombocytopenia (for all serious bleeding events, including intracranial hemorrhage [ICH] and meningitis (for ICH only). However, patients with severe thrombocytopenia and/or meningitis may be at greater risk for bleeding or ICH in the absence of drug therapy.

Immunomodulatory therapy

Corticosteroids have long been the subject of studies in sepsis, the rationale being that minimization of the inflammatory cascade could improve outcome. Short-term therapy with glucocorticoids has not improved outcomes in patients with sepsis, and a meta-analysis of 10 studies showed no beneficial effect [30]. A large scale, multicenter study is underway, but steroid therapy is not currently recommended in patients with sepsis.

Antibodies to TNF-α have been studied in sepsis, and, while most studies have found no benefit, one study showed a risk-adjusted relative reduction in mortality of 14.3% for septic patients with an IL-6 level of >1,000 pg/mL when treated with anti-TNF-α antibody [31].

Table 8. Causes of cardiogenic shock.

Causes of cardiogenic shock
Massive myocardial infarction
Small myocardial infarction in setting of reduced left ventricular function
Mitral regurgitation (due to papillary muscle rupture)
Rupture of interventricular septum
End stage cardiomyopathy
Myocarditis
Valvular heart disease
Hypertrophic cardiomyopathy

Studies have been carried out to evaluate the benefit in sepsis of anti-endotoxin, platelet activating factor antagonists, bradykinin antagonists, prostaglandin antagonists, IL-1 receptor antagonists, nonselective nitric oxide synthase inhibitors, *N*-acetyl cysteine, granulocyte colony-stimulating factor, and intravenous immunoglobulin G; none have been shown to be beneficial. A recent study assessing C1 inhibitor in 40 patients found an improvement in serum creatinine at days 3 and 4, but no survival benefit [32].

Hemofiltration in sepsis

Better understanding of the role of cytokines in sepsis and septic shock has led to the theory that removing them by hemofiltration may improve outcomes. Many studies have evaluated the effect of hemofiltration on cytokine levels and have shown that cytokines, including TNF-α, IL-1, IL-6, and IL-8 appear in the ultrafiltrate. While a few studies have shown a reduction in the amount of cytokines in the plasma with hemofiltration, the preponderance of studies have shown no reduction in plasma cytokine levels. The high production rate and rapid endogenous clearance of many cytokines mean that the amount being removed by hemofiltration is too minor to change circulating levels. It also appears that a large percentage of the clearance of cytokines occurs as a result of adsorption to the dialysis membrane, which soon becomes saturated, limiting further clearance.

In animal models, hemofiltration has improved survival in some studies, but these studies initiated hemofiltration before or shortly after the septic insult, which is generally not possible in clinical practice. Studies using a more realistic infection model have not shown an effect on survival. Prospective human studies to evaluate the benefit of hemofiltration in sepsis have generally been small. Reduction in the hyperdynamic response, including improved systemic vascular resistance, improvement in APACHE II scores, improvement in vasopressor requirement, and beneficial hemostatic changes have been found, but no randomized controlled trial has shown an improvement in survival when hemofiltration is used for sepsis.

Cardiogenic shock

Cardiogenic shock is defined as a state of decreased cardiac output in the setting of adequate intravascular volume that results in inadequate tissue perfusion. The diagnosis can be made clinically by finding signs of poor tissue perfusion, such as oliguria or cool extremities, along with the hemodynamic criteria of sustained hypotension (an SBP of <90 mm Hg), reduced cardiac index (<2.2 L/min/m^2), and congestion (a pulmonary capillary wedge pressure of

Table 9. Signs of cardiogenic shock.

Cardiac signs	Systemic signs (due to hypoperfusion)
Tachycardia	Confusion
Arrhythmias	Mottling of the skin
Jugular venous distention	Oliguria
Third heart sound	Pulmonary rales
	Lactic acidosis

>18 mm Hg). Cardiogenic shock occurs in 4.2%–7.2% of MIs and is the most common cause of death among patients suffering from MI, with a mortality rate of 60%. The most common cause of cardiogenic shock is massive MI; other causes are listed in **Table 8**.

Clinical features

Hypotension is universal in cardiogenic shock. Other common signs are shown in **Table 9**. Acute renal failure occurs in up to one-third of patients, and can increase mortality by 50%. Multiple organ failure develops in many patients, primarily due to ischemia from decreased cardiac output. However, high plasma levels of IL-6 have been associated with multiple organ failure in this population, indicating a possible role for systemic inflammation. Lactic acidosis may also occur from hypoperfusion.

Evaluation

The primary goal in the evaluation of cardiogenic shock is to determine the primary cause. While MI is the most common cause, other causes of shock, such as sepsis, hypovolemia, and pulmonary embolism, need to be considered. An ECG should be performed as soon as the patient arrives at the ICU, and, if an inferior MI is suspected, a right-sided ECG should be performed to evaluate for right-sided involvement. Routine blood tests (including assessment of cardiac enzymes) and a chest radiograph should be performed, and a Foley catheter should be placed to monitor urine output.

Echocardiography is a valuable tool for confirming the diagnosis of cardiogenic shock, and can evaluate potential mechanical causes that require surgical intervention, such as mitral regurgitation, papillary muscle rupture, tamponade, or left-ventricular free wall rupture.

Although assessment of brain natriuretic peptide (BNP) levels has been found to be effective in the diagnosis of congestive heart failure (CHF), it is not typically used in the diagnosis of cardiogenic shock. BNP levels have been found to decline as pulmonary capillary wedge pressure decreases, making BNP level a potential monitoring tool in the treatment of severe CHF, although it has not been extensively evaluated for cardiogenic shock.

Management

Airway management and maintenance of adequate oxygen supply should be the first concerns during resuscitation. Bi-level positive airway pressure or continuous positive airway pressure can improve oxygenation and avoid the need for intubation in patients with severe CHF, although their use in cardiogenic shock has not been intensively studied. Intubation and mechanical ventilation may be required if supplemental oxygen or noninvasive ventilation cannot maintain adequate oxygenation with minimal work of breathing.

Figure 2. Treatment of cardiogenic shock due to myocardial infarction.

ABG: arterial blood gas; CBC: complete blood count; ECG: electrocardiogram; IV: intravenous; NE: norepinephrine; NS: normal saline; Ntg: nitroglycerin; SBP: systolic blood pressure.

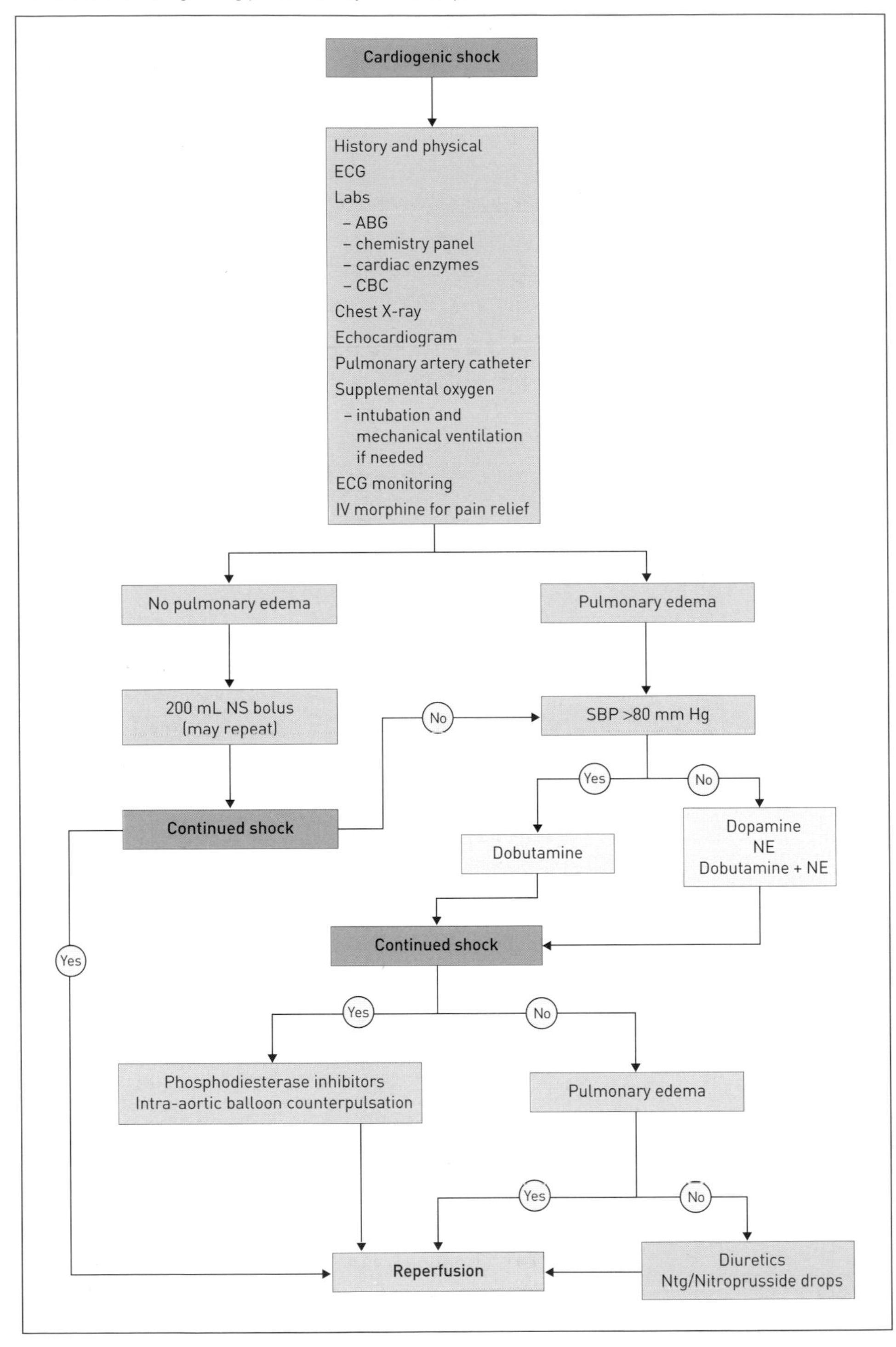

Patients treated for MI with β-blockers, angiotensin-converting enzyme (ACE) inhibitors, and nitrates who subsequently develop shock should have these agents discontinued as they may worsen the clinical state. Patients with mechanical causes of shock, such as valvular disease, should be evaluated for surgical repair.

Patients without a surgically treatable cause need aggressive medical therapy (see **Figure 2**). A minority of patients with cardiogenic shock may develop hypotension without evidence of pulmonary edema. In these patients, a fluid challenge of 100–250 mL of normal saline should be given to try and improve cardiac output. Inotropic agents should be administered to any patient who does not respond to fluids or has pulmonary congestion.

Dobutamine is primarily a β_1-adrenergic agonist, but is also a weak β_2- and α-adrenergic stimulator, and can improve myocardial contractility and cardiac output. Dobutamine is the drug of choice when SBP is >80 mm Hg, but can induce hypotension as a result of the β_2 effect, so should either not be used when blood pressure is <80 mm Hg or should be used in conjunction with another vasopressor. Dobutamine may worsen tachycardia and can cause arrhythmia.

Dopamine should be used when SBP is <80 mm Hg. At low doses (<5 μg/kg/min), β_1-adrenergic effects predominate; as the dose is increased, α-adrenergic effects prevail. However, patients vary in their responsiveness, and the lowest possible dose should be used. Norepinephrine is a pure α-adrenergic agonist and can be used when there is an inadequate response to dopamine.

Milrinone and amrinone are phosphodiesterase inhibitors that increase cyclic AMP levels in the myocardium. These agents increase inotropicity and cardiac output without increasing myocardial oxygen consumption. They do not induce direct tachycardia, but do cause peripheral vasodilatation, which can lead to hypotension and reflex tachycardia. As with dopamine and dobutamine, amrinone may improve myocardial mitochondrial function during shock.

If hemodynamics have stabilized after the initiation of vasopressors, the treatment of pulmonary edema with diuretics may be initiated. Direct vasodilator therapy can then be considered to decrease preload and afterload, which can improve ischemia. Sodium nitroprusside and nitroglycerin both have short half-lives, and can be carefully titrated, observing for worsening of the hemodynamic state.

Intra-aortic balloon pumping (IABP) can improve diastolic blood pressure, improve coronary perfusion, and increase cardiac output, and has been shown to improve in-hospital mortality [33]. IABP has a complication rate of 2%–15%, with a mortality rate of 0.05%–0.4%. Most of the complications are vascular, including major bleeding and limb ischemia; however, bacteremia and sepsis also occur.

The outcome of cardiogenic shock in the setting of MI is directly related to the patency of the involved coronary arteries. Therefore, the use of interventions to open occluded arteries is crucial. Thrombolytics can reduce mortality for patients in cardiogenic shock due to acute MI. However, recent evidence has favored an even more aggressive approach: revascularization by either percutaneous angioplasty or coronary artery bypass grafting should be considered in all

Table 10. Causes of hypertensive crises.

HELLP: hemolysis, elevated liver enzymes, and low platelets.

Idiopathic	Essential hypertension Malignant hypertension
Renal conditions	Acute glomerulonephritis Renal artery stenosis Vasculitis (polyarteritis nodosa, lupus) Scleroderma renal crisis Hemolytic-uremic syndrome/thrombocytopenic thrombotic purpura
Endocrine	Primary hyperaldosteronism Pheochromocytoma Cushing's syndrome
Drugs	Cocaine Amphetamines Clonidine withdrawal
Cardiovascular conditions	Coarctation of the aorta
Pregnancy related	Pre-eclampsia/eclampsia HELLP syndrome

patients with MI-induced cardiogenic shock. The administration of platelet glycoprotein IIb/IIIa inhibitor in conjunction with coronary stenting may further improve outcomes [34].

Ventricular assist devices have been used in peri-infarction cardiogenic shock, acute myocarditis, and postcardiotomy shock to bridge patients to either recovery of adequate myocardial function or transplantation.

Extracardiac obstructive shock

Several forms of shock are represented in this category, including pericardial tamponade-induced shock and pulmonary embolism-induced shock. During pericardial tamponade, shock can occur when increased pericardial pressure impairs the ability of the ventricle to fill during diastole, which results in decreased preload and cardiac output. Urgent pericardiocentesis and pericardiotomy are indicated. Pulmonary embolism can result in shock when a clot occludes more than 50%–60% of the pulmonary vascular bed. Left ventricular filling is drastically reduced with subsequent decreased cardiac output. In addition to heparin, thrombolytics can be used in the setting of massive pulmonary embolism with shock. Severe pulmonary hypertension can also result in shock.

Hypertensive crises

Hypertensive crises can be caused by several conditions (see **Table 10**). A hypertensive *emergency* occurs when elevated blood pressure (BP) is causing end-organ damage; this requires immediate therapy with parenteral antihypertensive agents. A hypertensive *urgency* occurs when there is markedly elevated BP without end-organ damage; this can be treated over several hours with oral antihypertensive agents. Malignant hypertension is present when the elevated BP is accompanied by papilledema (edema of the optic disc), retinal hemorrhage, or exudates.

End-organ damage in hypertensive emergencies is the result of a sequence of events. Vascular endothelial damage is caused by the mechanical stress of severe hypertension, leading to increased vascular permeability, as well as activation of the coagulation cascade. Microvascular thrombi formation can then occur, leading to ischemia. The

Table 11. Clinical findings in hypertensive emergencies.

Fundoscopic	Papilledema Hemorrhage Exudates
Neurologic	Confusion Seizures Headache Focal findings Somnolence Intracranial hemorrhage
Cardiac	Congestive heart failure Aortic dissection Acute myocardial infarction
Renal	Acute renal failure Proteinuria (may be nephrotic range) Hematuria
Hematologic	Microangiopathic hemolytic anemia
General	Malaise Nausea/vomiting

rennin–angiotensin–aldosterone system is upregulated, with angiotensin II causing vasoconstriction and potentiating the elevated BP.

Clinical findings

A markedly elevated BP is the most pertinent feature of malignant hypertension, but the absolute level does not correlate with symptoms. The rate of rise of BP is an important component, and a patient who was previously normotensive could have end-organ damage at a BP of 160/100, although most patients have a diastolic BP of >140 mm Hg. Other findings are listed in **Table 11**.

Evaluation

A patient presenting with a markedly elevated BP should receive a full history and physical, as well as a complete blood count, chemistry panel (to assess renal function and electrolytes), urinalysis, ECG, chest X-ray to evaluate for aortic dissection, and computed tomography scan of the brain if neurologic findings are present. If a secondary cause of hypertension is suspected (such as in someone younger than 30 years old, or someone who has a sudden onset of hypertension), plasma renin activity and aldosterone concentrations should be assessed to exclude primary hyperaldosteronism, a 24-hour urinalysis for metanephrines and catecholamines can assess for pheochromocytoma, and a magnetic resonance imaging study of the renal arteries can often identify renal artery stenosis. Women of child-bearing age should have a serum pregnancy test to rule out severe pre-eclampsia.

Treatment

Patients with evidence of end-organ damage due to hypertension should receive immediate therapy with parenteral agents, and the BP should be monitored with an arterial line. The initial decline in BP should be no more than 20%, or to approximately 160/110 (the decline should span 5–10 minutes for patients with acute aortic dissection, and 30–60 minutes for other patients). More rapid decreases in BP can lead to cerebral ischemia, since cerebral autoregulation is abnormal in many patients with malignant hypertension. After the initial decline, the BP can be further lowered over the next 2–3 days.

Table 12. Parenteral agents for hypertensive emergencies.

ACE: angiotensin-converting enzyme.

Drug	Dosage	Onset of action	Duration	Mechanism	Side effects
Nitroprusside	0.5–10 μg/kg/min	1–2 min	1–2 min	Arteriolar and venous dilator	Thiocyanate and cyanide toxicity
Nitroglycerin	5–100 μg/min	2–5 min	5–10 min	Reduces afterload and improves coronary artery perfusion	Methemoglobinemia
Hydralazine	10–20 mg bolus or 0.5–1 μg/min	1–5 min	3–6 h	Vasodilator	Reflex tachycardia, flushing
Labetalol	20–80 mg every 10 min, or 0.5 mg/min drops	5–10 min	2–6 h	α- and β-blocker with vasodilatory actions	Bradycardia, heart block
Esmolol	200–500 μg/kg for 1 min, then 50–300 μg/kg/min	1–2 min	10–30 min	β_1-selective β-blocker	Bradycardia Local skin necrosis if extravasates
Enalaprilat	0.6–5 mg every 6 h	5–15 min	6 h	ACE inhibitor	Acute renal failure
Nicardipine	5–15 mg/h	5–10 min	30 min	Calcium channel blocker	Tachycardia
Fenoldopam	0.1–0.6 μg/kg/min	4–5 min	10–15 min	D1 dopamine agonist	Reflex tachycardia Increased intraocular pressure

In patients with hypertensive urgency, BP can be lowered over 24–48 hours with oral medication.

Several agents are available for hypertensive emergencies (see **Table 12**). Nitroprusside is the drug of choice since it is a direct arteriolar and venous dilator with a rapid onset of action and short half-life, and therefore the dose can be rapidly titrated. Nitroprusside is metabolized to cyanide, which is rapidly metabolized to thiocyanate in the liver. Patients who receive this drug for several days may develop fatigue, nausea, and disorientation due to thiocyanate toxicity (>10 mg/dL), in which case nitroprusside treatment should be stopped. Cyanide toxicity can occur if the infusion rate is >20 μg/kg/min.

Nitroglycerin can reduce afterload and improve coronary artery perfusion, so is a first line agent in the setting of myocardial ischemia with a hypertensive emergency. However, it is not as reliable as nitroprusside, and tolerance can develop. Thus nitroglycerin should only be used as a second-line agent in other hypertensive emergencies.

Esmolol should be avoided in patients ingesting cocaine as the unopposed α-agonist effects of the cocaine can lead to worsening hypertension.

Enalaprilat (which produces enalapril) is an intravenous ACE inhibitor that can be used in the setting of congestive heart failure or scleroderma renal crisis.

The patient with a hypertensive urgency can usually be treated with oral agents. Sublingual nifedipine is to be avoided in these patients, as the acute drop in blood pressure can lead to myocardial or cerebral ischemia. If there is no clear cause for the elevated blood pressure, such as pain or anxiety, oral agents can be started. No single agent is considered

Table 13. Oral agents for the treatment of hypertensive urgency.

ACE: angiotensin-converting enzyme.

Drug	Dosage	Onset of action	Duration	Mechanism
Clonidine	0.2 mg initially, then 0.1 mg/h (up to 0.8 mg over 24 h)	30 min	6–8 h	Central α-adrenergic antagonist
Nifedipine	5–20 mg every 30 min	5–15 min	4–6 h	Calcium channel blocker
Nicardipine	20–40 mg every 8 h	30 min	8 h	Calcium channel blocker
Labetalol	100–400 mg every 2–4 h	0.5–2 h	8–12 h	α- and β-blocker
Captopril	12.5–50 mg every 8 h	30–90 min	4–6 h	ACE inhibitor

a drug of choice, but clonidine, nifedipine, and labetolol are most frequently used (see **Table 13**).

Pregnancy-related hypertensive crises

Severe hypertension and hypertensive encephalopathy can occur in pre-eclampsia. Pre-eclampsia is defined as the new onset of hypertension, proteinuria (>300 mg/day), and edema, usually occurring after 20 weeks gestation. Severe hypertension may occur at a lower BP than in non-pregnant paticnts, as thc vasodilatation during pregnancy normally results in a lower baseline BP. As in other hypertensive crises, the BP should be lowered by approximately 20% acutely, with hydralazine and labetalol considered first-line agents. Nitroprusside can be used in pregnancy, but cyanide and thiocyanate accumulation may occur in the fetus at doses >8 μg/kg/min. Nicardipine and clonidine may also be used. Refractory hypertension is an indication for delivery of the fetus. Other acute complications of pre-eclampsia include: eclampsia; hemolysis, elevated liver enzymes, low platelets (HELLP) syndrome; liver rupture; pulmonary edema; renal failure; DIC; and cortical blindness.

References

1. Bordin JO, Heddle NM, Blajchman MA. Biologic effects of leukocytes present in transfused cellular blood products. *Blood* 1994;84:1703–21.
2. Crosby ET. Perioperative hemotherapy: II. Risks and complications of blood transfusion. *Can J Anaesth* 1992;39:822–37.
3. Hebert PC, Wells G, Blajchman MA et al. A multicenter, randomized, controlled clinical trial of transfusion requirements in critical care. Transfusion Requirements in Critical Care Investigators, Canadian Critical Care Trials Group. *N Engl J Med* 1999;340:409–17. Erratum in: *N Engl J Med* 1999;340:1056.
4. Corwin HL, Gettinger A, Pearl RG et al. The CRIT study: anemia and blood transfusion in the critically ill – current clinical practice in the United States. *Crit Care Med* 2004;32:39–52.
5. Hebert PC, Wells G, Tweeddale M et al. Does transfusion practice affect mortality in critically ill patients? Transfusion Requirements in Critical Care (TRICC) Investigators and the Canadian Critical Care Trials Group. *Am J Respir Crit Care Med* 1997;155:1618–23.
6. Wu W-C, Rathore SS, Wang Y et al. Blood transfusion in elderly patients with acute myocardial infarction. *N Engl J Med* 2001;345:1230–6.
7. Hebert PC, Yetisir E, Martin C et al. Is a low transfusion threshold safe in critically ill patients with cardiovascular diseases? *Crit Care Med* 2001;29:227–34.
8. Rodriguez RM, Corwin HL, Gettinger A et al. Nutritional deficiencies and blunted erythropoietin response as causes of the anemia of critical illness. *J Crit Care* 2001;16:36–41.

9. Corwin HL, Gettinger A, Pearl RG et al. Efficacy of recombinant human erythropoietin in critically ill patients: a randomized controlled trial. *JAMA* 2002;288:2827–35.

10. Vincent JL. Plugging the leaks: new insight into synthetic colloids. *Crit Care Med* 1991;19:316–8.

11. Dahn MS, Lucas CE, Ledgerwood AM et al. Negative inotropic effect of albumin resuscitation for shock. *Surgery* 1979;86:235–41.

12. Lucas CE, Ledgerwood AM, Higgins RF. Impaired salt and water excretion after albumin resuscitation for hypovolemic shock. *Surgery* 1979;86:544–9.

13. Human albumin administration in critically ill patients: systematic review of randomised controlled trials. Cochrane Injuries Group Albumin Reviewers. *BMJ* 1998;317:235–40.

14. Schortgen F, Lacherade JC, Bruneel F et al. Effects of hydroxyethylstarch and gelatin on renal function in severe sepsis: a multicentre randomised study. *Lancet* 2001;357:911–6.

15. Thompson W. Rational use of albumin and plasma substitutes. *Johns Hopkins Med J* 1975;136:220–5.

16. Hollenberg S, Ahrens TS, Astiz ME et al. Practice parameters for hemodynamic support of sepsis in adult patients with sepsis. *Crit Care Med* 1999;22:639–60.

17. Malay MB, Ashton RC, Landry DW et al. Low-dose vasopressin in the treatment of vasodilatory septic shock. *J Trauma* 1999;47:699–703.

18. Jackson WL, Shorr AF. Vasopressin and cardiac performance. *Chest* 2002;121:1723–4.

19. Shapiro JI. Functional and metabolic responses of isolated hearts to acidosis: effects of sodium bicarbonate and Carbicarb. *Am J Physiol* 1990;258:H1835–9.

20. Arieff AI, Leach W, Park R et al. Systemic effects of $NaHCO_3$ in experimental lactic acidosis in dogs. *Am J Physiol* 1982;242:F586–91.

21. Tanaka M, Nishikawa T. Acute haemodynamic effects of sodium bicarbonate administration in respiratory and metabolic acidosis in anaesthetized dogs. *Anaesth Intensive Care* 1997;25:615–20.

22. Cooper D, Waller K, Wiggs B et al. Bicarbonate does not improve hemodynamics in critically ill patients who have lactic acidosis: a prospective, controlled clinical study. *Ann Int Med* 1990;112:492–8.

23. Mathieu D, Neviere R, Billard V et al. Effects of bicarbonate therapy on hemodynamics and tissue oxygenation in patients with lactic acidosis: a prospective, controlled clinical study. *Crit Care Med* 1991;19:1352–6.

24. Voelckel G, Lurie KG, Lindner KH et al. Vasopressin improves survival after cardiac arrest in hypovolemic shock. *Anesth Analg* 2000;91:627–34.

25. Angus DC, Linde-Zwirble WT, Lidicker J et al. Epidemiology of severe sepsis in the United States: analysis of incidence, outcome, and associated costs of care. *Crit Care Med* 2001;29:1303–10.

26. Marik PE, Varon J. Sepsis: state of the art. *Dis Mon* 2001;47:465–532.

27. Wheeler AP, Bernard GR. Current concepts: Treating patients with severe sepsis. *N Engl J Med* 1999;340:207–14.

28. Bernard GR, Vincent JL, Laterre PF et al. Efficacy and safety of recombinant human activated protein C for severe sepsis. *N Engl J Med* 2001;344:699–709.

29. Bernard GR, Macias WL, Joyce DE et al. Safety assessment of drotrecogin alfa (activated) in the treatment of adult patients with severe sepsis. *Crit Care* 2003;7:155–63.

30. Cronin L, Cook J, Carlet J et al. Corticosteroid treatment for sepsis: a critical appraisal and meta-analysis of the literature. *Crit Care Med* 1995;23:1430–9.

31. Pancek EA, Marshall J, Fishkoff S et al. Neutralization of tumor necrosis factor by a monoclonal antibody improves survival and reduces organ dysfunction in human sepsis: results of the MONARCS trial. *Chest* 2000;118:88S (Abstr.).

32. Caliezi C, Zeerleder S, Readondo M et al. C1 inhibitor in patients with severe sepsis and septic shock: beneficial effects on renal dysfunction. *Crit Care Med* 2002;30:1722–8.

33. Anderson RD, Ohman EM, Holmes DR et al. Use of intraaortic balloon counterpulsation in patients presenting with cardiogenic shock: observations from the GUSTO-I Study. Global Utilization of Streptokinase and TPA for Occluded Coronary Arteries. *J Am Coll Cardiol* 1997;30:708–15.

34. Tcheng JE. Glycoprotein IIb/IIIa receptor inhibitors: putting the EPIC, IMPACT II, RESTORE, and EPILOG trials into perspective. *Am J Cardiol* 1996;78(Suppl. 3A):35–40.

Section 2

Optimization

Part 1: Acid–base disorders

Richard N Hellman & Michael A Kraus

Approach to patients with an acid–base disorder

Acid–base disorders are frequently complex in intensive care unit patients and must be evaluated in a systematic manner. The acid–base disorders must be defined to help manage the patients' underlying disease processes, and care must be taken to avoid missing any aspect of a complex acid–base disorder.

Each time an acid–base disorder is encountered, the following seven questions should be answered:

1. Are there any life-threatening conditions?
2. Are the data correct?
3. What is the primary acid–base disturbance?
4. Is the degree of compensation appropriate?
5. How many different acid–base disturbances are present?
6. What is the differential diagnosis/etiology for each disorder?
7. What is the proper treatment?

Are there any life-threatening conditions?

Acid–base disorders can lead to life-threatening conditions. These conditions can be a direct result of acidosis – such as severe hypokalemia in a distal renal tubular acidosis – and usually represent electrolyte disorders, hemodynamic compromise, or hypoxia. A life-threatening condition may also be due to the etiology of the acid–base disorder – as is the case with ethylene glycol/methanol ingestion, or lactic acidosis secondary to septic shock or sepsis. Metabolic acidosis, metabolic alkalosis, respiratory acidosis, and respiratory alkalosis may also be life threatening if the disorder is particularly severe. These conditions must be immediately recognized and corrected to ensure proper treatment of the patient.

Are the data correct?

Serum bicarbonate is the most technically difficult electrolyte to measure and is the most likely to be incorrect on an electrolyte panel. An accurate serum bicarbonate measurement is essential as it helps determine the presence of an anion gap, and is necessary to determine the number of acid–base disturbances when they coexist. The accuracy of the measured serum bicarbonate level can be assessed using a manipulation of the Henderson–Hasselbach equation, where pCO_2 = partial pressure of CO_2:

$$[H^+] = (24)(pCO_2)/[HCO_3]$$

Table 1. Definitions of respiratory acidosis.

pCO_2: partial pressure of CO_2.

pCO_2	>40 mm Hg
pH	<7.35
Degree of compensation	
- Acute	pH increases by 0.08 for every 10 mm Hg fall in pCO_2 (no change in HCO_3)
- Chronic	pH increases by 0.03 for every 10 mm Hg fall in pCO_2 (HCO_3 increases 3-4mEq/L/10 mm Hg fall in pCO_2)
Metabolic acidosis	HCO_3<predicted

Table 2. Definitions of respiratory alkalosis.

pCO_2: partial pressure of CO_2.

pCO_2	<40 mm Hg
pH	>7.45
Degree of compensation	
- Acute	pH decreases by 0.08 for every 10 mm Hg rise in pCO_2 (HCO_3 decreases by 2-3 mEq/L/10 mm Hg rise in pCO_2)
- Chronic	pH decreases by 0.04 for every 10 mm Hg rise in pCO_2 (HCO_3 decreases by 4-5 mEq/L/10 mm Hg rise in pCO_2)
Metabolic alkalosis	HCO_3>predicted

To solve this equation for HCO_3, use the rearranged equation below:

$$[HCO_3] = (24)(pCO_2)/[H^+]$$

The H^+ concentration can be estimated by subtracting the last two digits (hundredths value) of the pH value from 80 when the pH is >7.0 and <7.55. For example, if the pH is 7.25 the hydrogen concentration can be estimated to be 80 minus 25. Alternatively, it can be calculated from the log of the pH. Many laboratories report the calculated HCO_3 with the arterial blood gas analysis (which provides the pCO_2); therefore, all variables in the equation should be available to assess whether the measured HCO_3 concentration is correct [1,2].

What is the primary acid–base disturbance?

Acidosis is the primary acid–base disturbance in the presence of acidemia (pH <7.35). The acidosis is termed "metabolic acidosis" if the bicarbonate is <24 mEq/mL and "primary respiratory acidosis" when the pCO_2 is greater than normal (40 mm Hg) (see **Table 1**).

Alkalosis always exists in the presence of alkalemia (pH>7.45). The alkalosis is termed "metabolic alkalosis" when the serum bicarbonate is >24 mEq/mL and "respiratory alkalosis" when it is secondary to hyperventilation and the pCO_2 is <40 mm Hg (see **Table 2**).

However, the physician must always remember to look at all the elements of an arterial blood gas analysis. A near normal pH is not sufficient evidence of a normal acid–base balance. pH can be normal in the presence of marked disturbances in bicarbonate and pCO_2, as is seen in the setting of a combined respiratory alkalosis and metabolic acidosis.

The answers to questions 4–7 are addressed in the following discussions of each disorder.

Table 3. Etiologies of respiratory acidosis and respiratory alkalosis.

CNS: central nervous system; COPD: chronic obstructive pulmonary disease.

Respiratory acidosis (hypoventilation)	CNS lesions Drug overdose/intoxication Anesthesia Primary respiratory failure (COPD/asthma) Potassium disorders Fatigue
Respiratory alkalosis (hyperventilation)	Aspirin intoxication Sepsis Hepatic failure Asthma/hypoxia Pulmonary embolus

Respiratory acid–base disturbances

A respiratory acidosis (also known as primary hypoventilation) can be considered primary when the pH is <7.40 and is accompanied by a rise in pCO_2 to a level >40 mm Hg (HCO_3 is usually ≥24 mEq/L). There is no change in HCO_3 concentration in acute respiratory acidosis, but after several hours or days, as the process becomes chronic, the kidney compensates with HCO_3 retention. In acute respiratory acidosis the pH decreases by 0.08 for every 10 mm Hg rise in pCO_2. In the chronic state, the kidney compensates for the acidosis and the HCO_3 increases by 3–4 mEq/L for every 10 mm Hg rise in pCO_2. Therefore, in the chronic state, the decrease in pH is only 0.03 for every 10 mm Hg rise in pCO_2 [1,2].

Conversely, in respiratory alkalosis (hyperventilation), the HCO_3 concentration decreases immediately (by 2–3 mEq/L) and the rise in pH is 0.08 for every 10 mm Hg fall in pCO_2. As the respiratory alkalosis persists, the kidney compensates; the HCO_3 decline increases to 4–5 mEq/L and the pH increase is only 0.04 for every 10 mm Hg fall in pCO_2.

The etiologies of respiratory acidosis and alkalosis are listed in **Table 3**. Treatment for these conditions consists of correction of the underlying disorder and correction of electrolyte and phosphorus disorders. Intubation and ventilation may become necessary to correct the ventilation, although this is more commonly required in respiratory acidosis than alkalosis.

Metabolic acidosis

The normal physiologic response to a primary metabolic acidosis (pH<7.40 and serum HCO_3 <24 mEq/L) is to increase ventilation, resulting in a decrease in pCO_2 and a rise in pH. This is termed the respiratory compensation to acidosis. A compensatory process, however, never fully or over compensates; in the setting of an acidosis the pH is always low. The degree of compensation or decrease in pCO_2 is similar in most patients for any degree of acidosis and can be estimated using the following equation [1,2]:

$$\mathbf{pCO_2 = (1.5 \times [HCO_3]) + 8 \pm 2}$$

If the measured pCO_2 is higher than the expected pCO_2 then a respiratory acidosis coexists with the metabolic acidosis. It is extremely important to recognize this as it may be the early presentation of impending respiratory failure, and elective intubation and ventilation may be indicated [1–3]. When the measured pCO_2 is less than the expected pCO_2, a respiratory alkalosis coexists with the metabolic acidosis. This may be a sign of early sepsis, aspirin intoxication, or relative hypoxia.

There is a useful shortcut for assessing respiratory compensation in the setting of metabolic acidosis (this is only applicable to metabolic acidosis). In the setting of appropriate respiratory compensation, the last two digits of the pH should be equal to the pCO_2. For example, when the pH is 7.21 the pCO_2 should be 21 mm Hg ± 2 mm Hg. Therefore, when the pCO_2 is greater than the last two digits of the pH, a respiratory acidosis coexists. When the pCO_2 is lower than the last two digits, a respiratory alkalosis coexists.

Anion gap metabolic acidosis

When determining the etiology and assessing whether more than one metabolic acidosis exists, the first step is to calculate the serum anion gap (SAG).

$$\mathbf{SAG = Na^+ - (Cl^- + HCO_3)}$$

A normal SAG is 8–12, but any value of <15 is satisfactory [4]. If the SAG is >15, an anion gap metabolic acidosis exists. The etiologies of anion gap metabolic acidosis are few and can be represented by the mnemonic MULEPAK: methanol, uremia, lactic acidosis, ethylene glycol, paraldehyde, aspirin, and ketosis (diabetic, alcoholic, starvation). To evaluate for the exact etiology, paraldehyde can be excluded; this is an old sedative and anticonvulsant not routinely used. Acidosis due to uremia, lactate, or ketosis can be easily recognized by detecting an elevated blood urea nitrogen (BUN) or creatinine (Cr), an arterial lactate level of >2.0 mEq/L, or the presence of serum ketones.

Treatment of uremia usually requires renal replacement therapy (RRT). If the uremia or the acidosis is not severe enough to warrant initiation of RRT then intravenous or enteral bicarbonate administration is indicated, as the uremic kidney is not able to generate bicarbonate.

Treatment of lactic acidosis requires recognition of the underlying cause and appropriately directed therapy (volume resuscitation, antibiotics, surgical resection of ischemic tissue). In cases of severe lactic acidosis, continuous RRT (see **Section 4**) can be used to stabilize the patient and allow medical and/or surgical interventions time to take effect and improve the patient's underlying disorder.

Ketosis is treated by increasing insulin levels. In the case of diabetic ketoacidosis, fluid resuscitation and insulin administration are indicated. In the absence of severe renal failure, aggressive potassium supplementation is also needed. Starvation and alcoholic ketoacidosis respond to the administration of glucose, provided the patient has the ability to secrete endogenous insulin. Supplementation with intravenous thiamine and folate is required when "feeding" the alcoholic patient.

Significant aspirin intoxication can usually be confirmed by history in the presence of tachycardia, diaphoresis, tremors, and, occasionally, respiratory alkalosis. When suspected, a serum aspirin level should be measured and, if elevated, treated with alkaline diuresis and/or hemodialysis. Hemodialysis is indicated when aspirin intoxication is associated with life-threatening complications or a serum aspirin level of >100 mg/dL.

Osmolar gap

Methanol and ethylene glycol are alcohols and may be ingested either intentionally or accidentally. Methanol may be found in a number of liquids, but is in high concentration in windshield solvent, and ethylene glycol is found in antifreeze. The patient may give a history of ingestion of these alcohols or may present with inebriation, confusion, or coma. They may present with heart failure, renal failure, and visual disturbances (with methanol) in the setting of a SAG metabolic acidosis. When suspected, serum methanol and ethylene glycol levels can be measured, although the appropriate technology is not always readily available. However, ingestion of either of these alcohols is always associated with an elevated osmolar gap.

$$\textbf{Osmolar gap} = \textbf{measured osmolality } (M_{OSM}) - \textbf{calculated osmolality } (C_{OSM})$$

$$C_{OSM} = 2[Na^+] + BUN/2.8 + Glucose/18 + Ethanol/4.6$$

An elevated osmolar gap (>15) in the setting of a SAG metabolic acidosis is indicative of ethylene glycol or methanol intoxication. Ethylene glycol intoxication can be confirmed by the presence of large calcium mono-oxalate crystals and blood in the urine. Treatment consists of either ethanol to maintain a blood-alcohol level of >100 mg/dL, or fomepizole at a dose of 15 mg/kg. If creatinine is not elevated and the HCO_3 level is >18 mEq/L then fomepizole can be continued on a 12-hourly basis. However, in most cases hemodialysis is indicated and care must be taken to maintain adequate ethanol or fomepizole levels during the hemodialysis session.

Combination metabolic acidosis

In the presence of an anion gap, always consider the possibility of the coexistence of an anion gap acidosis and a non-anion gap acidosis (hyperchloremic acidosis). In an anion gap acidosis, the anion gap will increase to the same degree that the HCO_3 concentration reduces, ie, for every 1 mEq/L decrease in HCO_3, the anion gap increases by 1. Therefore, the change in anion gap divided by the change in HCO_3 should be 1 [1–3]. This is termed the “delta/delta”:

$$\textbf{delta/delta} = \Delta_{AG}/\Delta_{HCO_3}$$

$$\Delta_{AG}/\Delta_{HCO_3} = \mathbf{1} \text{ (anion gap acidosis)}$$

$$\Delta_{AG}/\Delta_{HCO_3} \mathbf{<0.8} \text{ (suspect combination acidosis)}$$

Non-anion gap acidosis

The etiology of a non-anion gap acidosis is an acid ingestion, bicarbonate loss, or an inability to excrete an acid load (see **Table 4**). To determine the etiology of a non-anion gap acidosis,

Table 4. Etiology of non-anion gap (hyperchloremic) acidosis.

DKA: diabetic ketoacidosis; RTA: renal tubular acidosis.

Acid infusions	Bicarbonate losses	Inability to secrete acid
Amino acid Hydrochloric acid Re-expansion acidosis Ammonium chloride	Gastrointestinal: – diarrhea – enterocutaneous fistula – transplanted pancreas (with bladder anastomosis) Renal: – proximal RTA (type II RTA) – carbonic anhydrase inhibitor – DKA recovery	Distal RTA (type I RTA) Type IV RTA Renal failure

Table 5. Evaluation of non-anion gap (hyperchloremic) acidosis.

GI: gastrointestinal; RTA: renal tubular acidosis.

[a]Can be much lower in Fanconi's syndrome; [b]in steady state or under acid load, will be elevated if bicarbonate is administered; [c]variable, depends on degree of GI losses or when RTA is identified, may be <10.

	GI losses	Distal RTA	Proximal RTA	Type IV RTA
Potassium	Low	Low	Low	High
Bicarbonate	Variable	Variable	18–21[a]	18–21
Urine pH	<5.5	>5.5	<5.5[b]	<5.5
Urine anion gap	Negative	Positive	Negative	Positive[c]

measure the serum K^+, serum HCO_3, urine pH, and the urine anion gap (UAG) (see **Table 5**):

$$\mathbf{UAG = Na^+ + K^+ - Cl^-}$$

The UAG is positive at baseline and becomes negative in metabolic acidosis associated with a functioning distal tubule (when protons can be secreted) [5] and NH_4Cl is the titratable acid. In order to allow for the secretion of protons in the distal tubule, protons need to be buffered to prevent lowering of the pH to a level that turns off proton secretion. While phosphates and sulfates are excellent buffers at this pH, they are not readily present in sufficient quantity to allow adequate buffering. NH_3 is the buffer available in the distal tubule as it is generated in the proximal tubule and stored in the medulla. NH_3 is secreted into the thick ascending limb and, in the absence of protons, it is reabsorbed back into the medulla. In the presence of free protons ammonium is created and trapped in the distal tubule because ammonium ions cannot be reabsorbed. Hence, NH_4Cl is the titratable acid readily available in the distal tubule. As NH_4Cl is secreted, the chloride concentration in the urine increases and the urinary anion gap becomes negative [5–7].

In the setting of gastrointestinal (GI) HCO_3 losses or acid infusions, the kidney functions normally and the distal tubule is able to secrete a titratable acid (NH_4Cl); the proximal tubule reabsorbs bicarbonate; ammonia is available; and the distal tubule can secrete protons via the H^+ ATPase. Therefore, K^+ is low due to losses through the GI tract, urinary pH is appropriately acidic, and the UAG is negative. With GI etiologies of non-anion gap acidosis,

Table 6. Common causes of renal tubular acidosis (RTA).

Distal RTA (type I)	Proximal RTA (type II)	Type IV RTA
Congenital	Disorders of metabolism	Hyporenin, hypoaldosterone state
Disorders of metabolism	Heavy metal intoxication	Elderly diabetic
Amyloidosis	Nephrotic syndrome	Interstitial nephritis from any cause
Hypercalcemic states	Carbonic anhydrase inhibitors	
Toluene/amphotericin B		

treatment consists of control of the GI losses and adequate hydration with K^+ supplementation as indicated. If the acidosis is due to acid ingestion, discontinue the source. In the case of acidosis due to hyperalimentation, adding acetate or lactate to the total parenteral nutrition prescription will correct the acidosis.

In the case of proximal renal tubular acidosis [8], there are multiple potential etiologies that lead to the loss of HCO_3 in the proximal tubule and an inability to reabsorb HCO_3 (see **Table 6**). In the steady state situation or during acid loading, the distal tubule can secrete an acid load. The presence of an acidosis stimulates aldosterone release, and Na^+ and K^+ channels are opened in the distal tubule. Therefore, there is urinary loss of K^+ and serum levels are correspondingly low. The urine pH is appropriately acidic and the UAG should be negative. With the exception of Fanconi's syndrome, the acidosis in proximal tubular acidosis is not associated with significant morbidity and is generally not severe. Therefore, treatment of the acidosis is generally not indicated. This is fortunate because the alkali requirement to correct this disorder is very large (10–20 mEq/kg/day) due to the large amounts required to overcome the urinary losses of HCO_3 as its concentration rises.

Distal renal tubular acidosis is associated with significant morbidity. Nephrocalcinosis, nephrolithiasis, and bone disease are common sequelae of prolonged distal renal tubular acidosis. The etiology of these disorders is damage to the distal tubule leading to the inability to secrete an acid load and generate HCO_3. The distal tubule is responsible for the generation of 1–2 mEq/kg/day of HCO_3 to balance the daily acid generation and load. Without the ability to secrete acids and generate HCO_3 in the distal tubule, patients become progressively acidotic. Over time they can become severely acidotic, with serum HCO_3 concentrations below 10 mEq/L. The acidosis stimulates aldosterone and this leads to the opening of distal tubule sodium and potassium channels leading to urinary K^+ loss and hypokalemia. Since the distal tubule cannot secrete protons in the setting of a distal renal tubular acidosis, the urinary pH remains elevated (>6.0) and NH_4Cl cannot be generated/secreted. This leads to a high urinary pH for the degree of acidosis and a positive urinary anion gap. Hence patients with distal renal tubule acidosis are hypokalemic, variably acidotic, unable to generate acid urine, and have a positive urinary anion gap. Treatment of this disorder consists of correction of the underlying cause and supplementation of alkali and K^+. Citrate solutions are available that contain 1 mEq of sodium citrate and 1 mEq of potassium citrate per mL. Patients who receive these solutions usually respond to a dose of 2 mEq/kg/day given in divided doses. In patients with bone disease, supplementation with vitamin D may also be beneficial.

The etiology of type IV renal tubular acidosis is a hyporenin, hypoaldosterone state [8]. This condition often occurs in diabetic patients who have little or no renal dysfunction [9]. In this condition, the juxtaglomerular apparatus does not generate renin. In the absence of renin, angiotensin I is not converted to angiotensin II, which is the major stimulus for aldosterone production. Therefore, aldosterone is not generated or secreted in the hyporenin state. In the absence of aldosterone, the distal tubule does not stimulate distal sodium reabsorption (decreased Na^+/K^+ ATPase and Na^+ channel activity) nor does it secrete sufficient K^+ (decreased activity of K^+ channels). Interestingly, the activity of the H^+ ATPase is usually normal; therefore, serum K^+ rises, which is the hallmark of type IV RTA. This rise in serum K^+ leads to intracellular exchange of K^+ for H^+, thus decreasing the pH of the extracellular fluid (ECF). In addition, hyperkalemia inhibits the activity of the enzymes responsible for ammoniagenesis in the renal proximal tubule. The lack of ammoniagenesis leads to the loss of the medullary ammonia gradient and an inability to buffer and secrete an acid load. To summarize, K^+ is elevated, HCO_3 is moderately depressed (18–21 mEq/L), and the urine has an acid pH (<5.5) with a positive UAG and an inability to secrete ammonium chloride. The treatment of type IV RTA consists of lowering serum K^+; administration of alkali is unnecessary. Treatment with loop diuretics will lower K^+, which is particularly useful in the setting of hypertension, mild fluid overload, history of pulmonary edema, or renal insufficiency. However, loop diuretics are potentially harmful in the setting of significant orthostatic hypotension. K^+ can also be lowered with use of a mineral-ocorticoid supplement (fludrocortisone [Florinef; Monarch Pharmaceuticals, Bristol, TN, USA] 0.1 mg/day). Fludrocortisone is useful in the setting of orthostatic hypotension but contraindicated in fluid retention states and difficult-to-control hypertension.

Metabolic alkalosis

Metabolic alkalosis is a primary acid–base disturbance due to either loss of acid (H^+) or gain of HCO_3 in the ECF. In this condition, the blood has a pH of >7.4 and plasma HCO_3 of >26–28 mEq/L [10,11]. Metabolic alkalosis occurs in half of all patients hospitalized with an acid–base disorder [10,11]. A direct relationship between mortality and blood pH exists when the blood pH is >7.48. Mortality rates of 45% and 80% have been noted at blood pH levels of 7.55 and 7.65, respectively [10,11]. Metabolic alkalosis may be a marker rather than a cause of mortality. Major adverse effects of alkalemia are frequently seen when blood pH is ≥7.6 [10–13].

Renal HCO_3 management

An HCO_3 load is initially managed by extracellular and intracellular buffering. Eighty-five percent of the filtered load of HCO_3 is reabsorbed in the proximal tubule: 10% in the thick ascending limb, and 5% in the cortical collecting duct and inner medullary collecting duct. The kidney has the ability to reabsorb all plasma HCO_3 below a level of 26–28 mEq/L and to excrete all HCO_3 when the plasma HCO_3 is above this level. This level is called the HCO_3 threshold or tubular maximum for bicarbonate (Tm HCO_3) (see **Figure 1**) [12,14].

Factors affecting renal HCO_3 reabsorption include ECF volume, pCO_2, serum K^+, and mineralocorticoids (see **Table 7**) [10,12,14]. In the presence of ECF volume contraction,

Figure 1. Filtration, reabsorption, and excretion of bicarbonate as functions of plasma concentration in normal subjects.

Reproduced with permission from Pitts RF (RFP), Ayer JL (JLA), Schiess WA (WAS). *J Clin Invest* 1949;28:35.

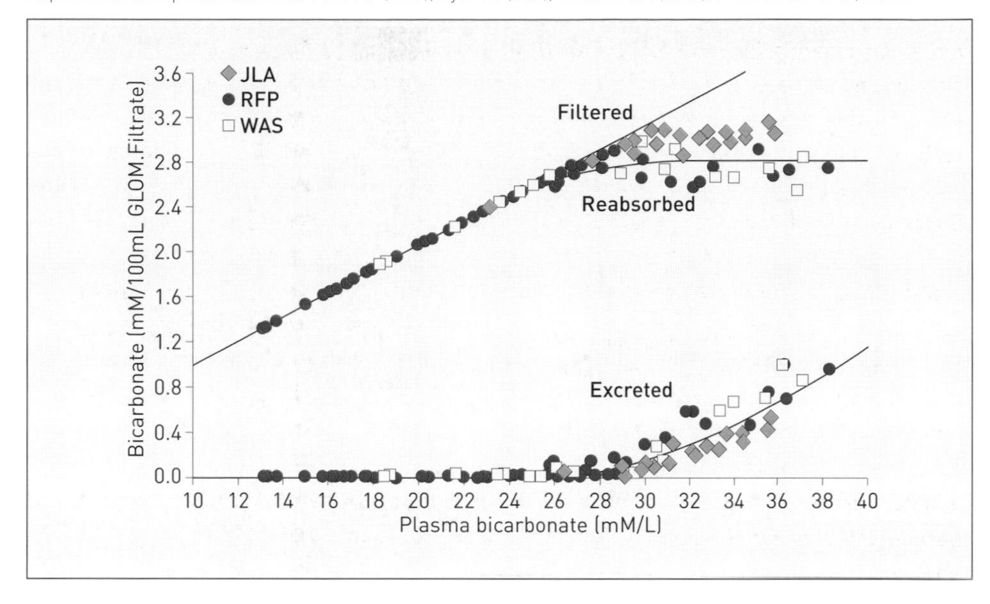

Table 7. Factors affecting renal HCO_3 reabsorption (H^+ secretion).

ECF: extracellular fluid.

Increasing	Decreasing
ECF volume contraction	ECF volume expansion
Hypercapnia	Hypocapnia
K^+ depletion	K^+ excess
Mineralocorticoid excess	Mineralocorticoid depletion

hypercapnia, hypokalemia, or mineralocorticoid excess, renal H^+ secretion and serum HCO_3 reabsorption are increased [10].

Generation and maintenance of metabolic alkalosis

Onset of vomiting with ECF volume contraction can be associated with activation of the renin–angiotensin–aldosterone system and hypokalemia. The generation of metabolic alkalosis due to loss of hydrochloric acid from the stomach alone is not enough to sustain metabolic alkalosis; it is sustained by secondary hyperaldosteronism, chloride depletion, and hypokalemia. Similarly, the infusion of $NaHCO_3$ alone will not sustain metabolic alkalosis – due to the HCO_3 threshold – unless a maintaining factor such as K^+ depletion, ECF volume contraction, mineralocorticoid excess, or hypercapnia is present [10–12,14].

Metabolic alkalosis occurs as a result of either net acid loss or net alkali gain, and may result from renal or extrarenal causes. However, this may not be sufficient to sustain metabolic alkalosis; the maintenance of metabolic alkalosis is due either to impaired renal HCO_3 excretion or enhanced renal HCO_3 reabsorption. The concept of the generation and

Table 8. Generation of metabolic alkalosis.

NG: nasogastric; V: vomiting.

Reproduced with permission from Palmer BF, Alpern RJ. Metabolic alkalosis. *J Am Soc Nephrol* 1997;8:1462–9.

Extrarenal	Renal
Excessive acid loss: - loss in gastric juice. V, NG suction - intestinal loss: villous - adenoma, congenital - chloridorrhea Translocation into cells: - Na^+ deficiency Excessive gain of HCO_3: - oral or parenteral HCO_3 intake - metabolism of lactate, ketones, or other organic anions to HCO_3	Coupling of high mineralocorticoid activity and high distal Na^+ delivery Mineralocorticoid excess K^+ deficiency

Table 9. Maintenance of metabolic alkalosis.

EAV: effective arterial blood volume; ECF: extracellular fluid; GFR: glomerular filtration rate.

Increased proximal HCO_3 reabsorption	Increased distal HCO_3 reabsorption	Decreased nephron mass
Increased H^+ secretion	Mineralocorticoid excess	Chronic kidney disease
Decreased EAV (ECF volume contraction)	Hypokalemia	Decreased GFR
Hypercapnea	Chloride depletion	
Hypokalemia	Non-reabsorbable anion	
Hypoparathyroidism		
Hypercalcemia		

maintenance of metabolic alkalosis is critical to the understanding of this condition. The factors that contribute to the generation and maintenance of metabolic alkalosis are listed in **Tables 8** and **9** [11,12].

Respiratory compensation for metabolic alkalosis consists of hypoventilation with a subsequent increase in pCO_2. This can be of clinical significance in patients with underlying chronic obstructive pulmonary disease (COPD), where an increase in serum HCO_3 due to diuretics can cause hypoventilation and respiratory failure [13,15,16]. In the absence of pulmonary disease, pCO_2 rarely exceeds 55 mm Hg. Formulae that can be used to calculate the degree of respiratory compensation for metabolic alkalosis are listed in **Table 10**.

Electrolyte patterns in metabolic alkalosis include a normal serum Na^+, which can be reduced in diuretic therapy; hypokalemia; an elevated serum HCO_3; and a low serum chloride (hypokalemic, hypochloremic metabolic alkalosis).

The anion gap in metabolic alkalosis is usually normal or only minimally increased. However, metabolic alkalosis with volume depletion can raise the anion gap by 5 mEq/L for each 0.1 increase in pH. This is due to increased serum albumin concentration, a

Table 10. Calculating respiratory compensation for metabolic alkalosis.

pCO_2: partial pressure of CO_2.

Clinical pearl	pCO_2 is rarely ≥55 mm Hg except with primary pulmonary disease
Clinical pearl	pCO_2 increase is variable
Formula 1	$pCO_2 = 0.9[HCO_3] + 9$
Formula 2	pCO_2 increases by 0.6 mm Hg for each 1 mEq/L increase in HCO_3

Table 11. Major adverse consequences of severe alkalemia (pH≥7.6).

Reproduced with permission from Adrogué HJ, Madias NE. Management of life-threatening acid–base disorders. Second of two parts. *N Engl J Med* 1998;338:107–11.

Cardiovascular	Arteriolar constriction Reduction in coronary blood flow Reduction in anginal threshold Predisposition to refractory supraventricular and ventricular arrhythmias
Cerebral	Reduction in cerebral blood flow Tetany, seizures, lethargy, delirium, and stupor
Respiratory	Hypoventilation with attendant hypercapnia and hypoxemia
Metabolic	Stimulation of anaerobic glycolysis and organic acid production Hypokalemia Decreased plasma ionized calcium concentration Hypomagnesemia and hypophosphatemia

pH-dependent increase in the negative charge on albumin, and stimulation of 6-phosphofructokinase with increased serum lactate and ketone production [15,17,18].

The major adverse consequences of severe alkalemia (pH>7.6) are shown in **Table 11**. Respiratory depression and decreased oxygen delivery due to vasoconstriction and the Bohr effect occur with severe metabolic alkalosis. The cardiac effects of metabolic alkalosis include reduction in coronary artery blood flow, a reduced anginal threshold, and a predisposition to refractory ventricular and supraventricular arrhythmias. Cerebral blood flow is reduced due to vasoconstriction, which may lead to tetany, seizures, altered sensorium, and coma. Stimulation of anaerobic glycolysis, hypokalemia, decreased ionized calcium, hypocalcemia, and hypophosphatemia can occur as a result of metabolic alkalosis [10,11,13,14].

Syndromes of metabolic alkalosis can be divided into those disorders associated with volume contraction, volume expansion, renal insufficiency, or severe potassium deficiency (see **Table 12**).

Management approach to metabolic alkalosis

An approach to the patient with metabolic alkalosis is shown in **Figure 2** [11]. Evaluation of the patient's volume status and the presence or absence of hypertension or hypotension is critical. A history of diuretic, cathartic, or sodium bicarbonate use, or milk-alkali syndrome, should be obtained. It is important to obtain a thorough family history to evaluate for disorders such as Bartter's syndrome or Gitelman's syndrome.

Table 12. Syndromes of metabolic alkalosis.

BP: blood pressure; DOC: deoxycorticosterone; ECF: extracellular fluid; GFR: glomerular filtration rate; GI: gastrointestinal; NG: nasogastric; RAS: renal artery stenosis.

Reproduced with permission from Palmer BF, Alpern RJ. Metabolic alkalosis. *J Am Soc Nephrol* 1997;8:1462–9.

Effective volume contraction	Secondary hyperaldosteronism; BP normal or low
GI, dietary, or other non-renal generation	Vomiting; NG suction; Cl^- wasting diarrhea; villous adenoma; contraction alkalosis; K^+ deficiency
Renal generation	Diuretics; volume depletion; increased distal delivery of poorly reabsorbable anions; Bartter's syndrome; Gitelman's syndrome; post-hypercapnia; magnesium deficiency and hypercalcemia of malignancy
ECF volume expansion with mineralocorticoid effect	BP increased
Increased renin and aldosterone	RAS; accelerated hypertension; renin-secreting tumor
Decreased renin, increased aldosterone	Primary aldosteronism; adrenal adenoma; bilateral adrenal hyperplasia; dexamethasone-responsive adrenal hyperplasia; carcinoma
Decreased renin, decreased aldosterone	Cushing's syndrome; exogenous mineralocorticoid; congenital adrenal enzyme defect; 11β and 17α hydroxylase deficiency (DOC and corticosterone); Liddle's syndrome; licorice (glycyrrhic acid)
Renal insufficiency	Exogenous HCO_3 load in the setting of decreased GFR; milk-alkali syndrome; plasmapheresis (sodium citrate load); orthotopic liver transplantation (citrate load)

Figure 2. Approach to the patient with metabolic alkalosis.

A: aldosterone; ABC: airway-breathing-circulation; ABG: arterial blood gases; EAV: effective arterial blood volume; FENa: fractional excretion of sodium; R: renin; U: urinary.

[a]See **Table 12**.

Reproduced with permission from Palmer BF, Alpern RJ. Metabolic alkalosis. *J Am Soc Nephrol* 1997;8:1462–9.

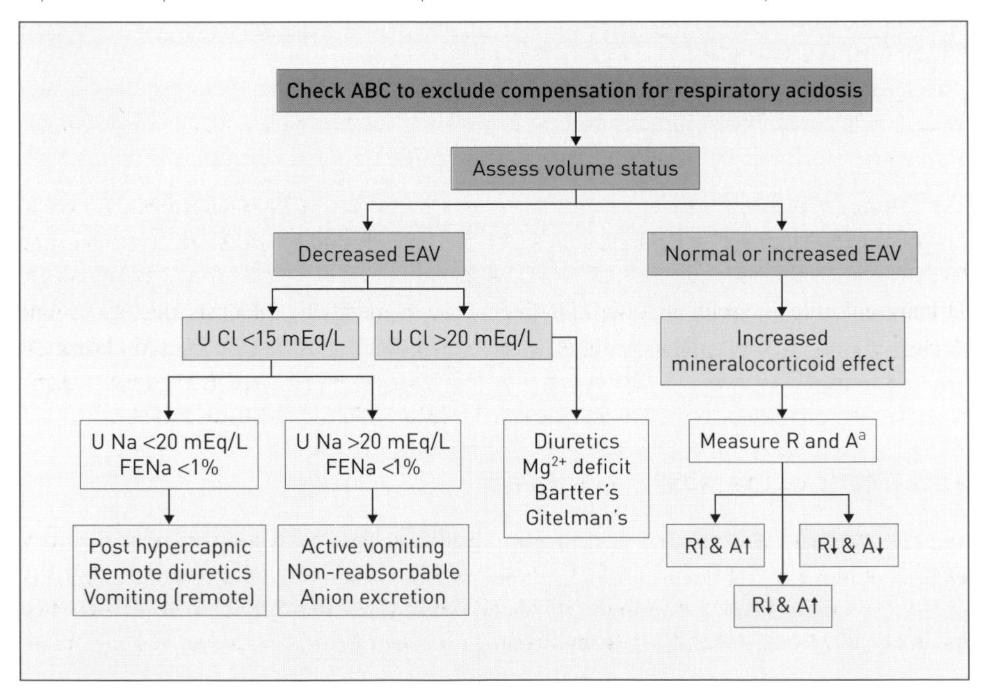

Table 13. Differential diagnosis of metabolic alkalosis with urinary chloride (U Cl^-).

GI: gastrointestinal.

Reprinted from *Primer on Kidney Diseases*, Second Edition, Jones ER. Chapter 10: Metabolic alkalosis: 80–5. Copyright 2004, with permission from Elsevier.

U Cl^- <15 mEq/L (Cl^- responsive)	U Cl^- >20 mEq/L (Cl^- resistant)
GI fluid loss	Primary aldosteronism
Stool loss (Cl^- losing diarrhea)	Exogenous steroids
Diuretics (screen negative/remote diurectic use)	Diuretics (recent)
Post-hypercapnia	Bartter's syndrome or Gitelman's syndrome
Refeeding	Cushing's syndrome
Low Cl^- intake	Alkali loading
Cystic fibrosis	Hypercalcemia
	Hypomagnesemia
	Severe hypokalemia

Table 14. Treatment of chloride-responsive metabolic alkalosis.

CVVH: continuous venovenous hemofiltration; CVVHD: continuous venovenous hemodialysis; EAV: effective arterial volume; GI: gastrointestinal; NS: normal saline; PD: peritoneal dialysis; PO: orally; IV: intravenously.

Decreased EAV
NaCl volume expansion with NS
KCl (PO or IV)
Discontinuance of diuretics
Mg^{2+} repletion in Mg^{2+} depletion (PO or IV)
Acetazolamide
Hemodialysis, CVVH, CVVHD, or PD
HCl (IV, central vein)
Decrease gastric acid production if GI loss:
- proton pump inhibitor
- H_2 blocker
NH_4Cl (IV peripheral vein)

Laboratory evaluation should include serum creatinine, BUN, electrolytes, calcium, phosphorus, magnesium, and albumin. A spot urine test for chloride, sodium, creatinine, and fractional excretion of sodium, and a complete blood count (CBC) should be obtained. Urinary chloride is useful in discriminating between metabolic alkalosis due to volume depletion and metabolic alkalosis due to mineralocorticoid or mineralocorticoid-like excess syndromes (see **Table 13**) [11,12]. In patients with normal or increased EAV hypertension, measurement of plasma renin and aldosterone levels is indicated in **Figure 2** [11].

Treatment of metabolic alkalosis

General principles of treatment for metabolic alkalosis include correction of volume deficits, potassium and/or magnesium deficits, and prevention of continued losses [10,11,13]. Treatment can be divided into that for chloride-responsive and that for chloride-resistant metabolic alkalosis [10,12,14]. It is important to conduct follow-up tests of volume status,

Table 15. Treatment of chloride-resistant metabolic alkalosis.

ACE: angiotensin-converting enzyme; ARB: angiotensin receptor blocker; NSAID: nonsteroidal anti-inflammatory drug.

Mineralocorticoid excess	Spironolactone Possible surgery if adenoma
Liddle's syndrome	Amiloride (5–10 mg/day)
Bartter's syndrome and Gitelman's syndrome	KCl High K^+ diet ACE inhibitors or ARB NSAID Correction of magnesium depletion K^+-sparing diuretics: amiloride, triamterene, spironolactone

intake and output, daily weight, serum, creatinine, BUN, electrolytes, calcium, phosphorus, glucose, and pH both during and after treatment.

Treatment of chloride-responsive metabolic alkalosis

The treatment strategies for chloride-responsive metabolic alkalosis are shown in **Table 14**. Isotonic saline is the first step in therapy. The patient usually requires 3–5 L of 0.9% NaCl over the first 24 hours. Chloride repletion is important for the correction of metabolic alkalosis. Chloride depletion can be thought of as being synonymous with volume depletion. Chloride is necessary for tubular reabsorption of sodium and to minimize the exchange of sodium for hydrogen, which favors bicarbonate generation and distal tubule chloride reabsorption with bicarbonate excretion. The total body chloride deficit (BCD) can be calculated using the following formula:

$$\mathbf{BCD = (0.2)(body\ weight\ in\ kg)(change\ in\ plasma\ Cl^-)}$$

The change in plasma chloride can be calculated by subtracting the measured plasma chloride from the desired plasma chloride. Potassium chloride needs to be repleted. Maintenance doses of 20 mEq/L of potassium chloride in normal saline should be used in addition to correcting potassium deficits. Metabolic alkalosis is usually hypokalemic metabolic alkalosis. Giving normal saline alone will cause increased distal tubular sodium reabsorption and potassium secretion leading to hypokalemia. (See **Treatment of hypokalemia**, *page 98*). Diuretics should be discontinued or their dosages reduced. Magnesium repletion is necessary in the presence of hypomagnesemia. Care should be taken in metabolic alkalosis patients with renal insufficiency. Acetazolamide can be used at doses of 250–500 mg/day to reduce serum HCO_3 if there is adequate renal function (a serum creatinine level of <4 mg/dL) and no acidosis. Metabolic acidosis, bicarbonaturia, and hypokalemia are potential complications of acetazolamide therapy and need to be carefully monitored. In the presence of increased gastric acid loss, proton pump inhibitors and/or H_2 blockers are helpful in reducing gastric acid loss [10,11]. The majority of cases of chloride-resistant metabolic alkalosis respond to normal saline KCl and/or acetazolamide.

Hemodialysis, peritoneal dialysis, or continuous renal replacement therapies can be used for the correction of severe chloride-responsive metabolic alkalosis that is not responsive to medical therapy, or severe chloride-responsive metabolic alkalosis in the presence of renal failure. Hemodialysis requires a low concentration HCO_3 bath, since the usual hemodialysis bath contains 35 mEq/L of HCO_3; peritoneal dialysis using sterile normal saline with appropriate potassium, calcium, and magnesium replacement can also be utilized. Where available, acute hemodialysis is the preferred treatment modality due to its ability to rapidly correct metabolic alkalosis [10,11,19].

Ammonium chloride (at an infusion rate of <300 mEq/day) has been used to treat chloride-responsive metabolic alkalosis but is contraindicated in patients with hepatic or renal disease. It can be given intravenously via a peripheral vein. Hydrochloric acid (HCl) may be given to patients with chloride-responsive severe metabolic alkalosis (pH>7.55) if other therapies have failed and the patient has hepatic encephalopathy, cardiac arrhythmia, altered mental status, or digitalis intoxication. HCl use is complicated by the need for central line placement with position verification. Tissue necrosis is a severe side effect of extravasation and must be avoided. HCl should only be used by those experienced in this therapy. Hemodialysis is, in this author's opinion, a preferred alternative to HCl. If HCl is used, the desired deficit of acid needs to be calculated. This can be done using the following equation:

$$\textbf{Desired deficit of acid} = \textbf{(0.5)(body weight in kg)(the desired decrement in } \mathbf{HCO_3}\textbf{)}$$

The object of therapy is to restore half of the normal HCO_3 excess over 24 hours. The infusion rate of HCl should be <25 mEq/h. HCl has been added to total parenteral nutrition solutions [10,11].

Treatment of chloride-resistant metabolic alkalosis

The treatment strategies for chloride-resistant metabolic alkalosis are shown in **Table 15**. The first step in the treatment of this disorder is to address the underlying condition. Magnesium levels need to be repleted if hypokalemia or hypomagnesemia is present.

Mineralocorticoid excess syndromes, such as hyperaldosteronism, should be treated with spironolactone (25–50 mg four times a day). Primary hyperaldosteronism warrants surgical treatment in suitable candidates with adrenal adenoma.

Bartter's syndrome and Gitelman's syndrome pose a particular challenge in the management of chloride-resistant hypokalemic metabolic alkalosis. The repletion of potassium requires KCl in addition to the use of high-potassium foods (see **Treatment of hypokalemia**, *page 98*). Angiotensin converting enzyme inhibitors and angiotensin receptor blockers can be useful in maintaining normokalemia. The use of nonsteroidal anti-inflammatory drugs is occasionally helpful. Correction of magnesium depletion and use of potassium-sparing diuretics, particularly amiloride, may also be of value. Oral amiloride at doses of 5–10 mg/day, oral triamterene at 100 mg twice daily, or oral spironolactone at 25–50 mg four times a day are helpful as potassium-sparing diuretics. Hyperkalemia related to treatment needs to be monitored.

References

1. Rose B, Narins R, Post T, editors. *Clinical Physiology of Acid–Base and Electrolyte Disorders*. New York, NY: McGraw-Hill, Inc., 1994.

2. Narins RG, Emmett M. Simple and mixed acid–base disorders: a practical approach. *Medicine (Baltimore)* 1980;59:161–87.

3. Adrogue HJ, Madias NE. Management of life-threatening acid–base disorders. First of two parts. *N Engl J Med* 1998;338:26–34.

4. Emmett M, Narins RG. Clinical use of the anion gap. *Medicine (Baltimore)* 1977;56:38–54.

5. Batlle DC, Hizon M, Cohen E et al. The use of the urinary anion gap in the diagnosis of hyperchloremic metabolic acidosis. *N Engl J Med* 1988;318:594–9.

6. Dyck RF, Asthana S, Kalra J et al. A modification of the urine osmolar gap: an improved method for estimating urine ammonium. *Am J Nephrol* 1990;10:359–62.

7. Kamel KS, Ethier JH, Richardson RM et al. Urine electrolytes and osmolality: when and how to use them. *Am J Nephrol* 1990;10:89–102.

8. Smulders YM, Frissen PH, Slaats EH et al. Renal tubular acidosis. Pathophysiology and diagnosis. *Arch Intern Med* 1996;156:1629–36.

9. Uribarri J. Acid–base Considerations in Renal Failure. *Semin Dial* 2000;13:211–70.

10. Galla JH. Metabolic alkalosis. *J Am Soc Nephrol* 2000;11:369–75.

11. Palmer BF, Alpern RJ. Metabolic alkalosis. *J Am Soc Nephrol* 1997;8:1462–9.

12. Jones ER. Metabolic Alkalosis. In: Greenburg A, Coffman TM, editors. *Primer on Kidney Diseases*. 3rd ed. Amsterdam: Academic Press, 2001:81–6.

13. Adrogue HJ, Madias NE. Management of life-threatening acid–base disorders. Second of two parts. *N Engl J Med* 1998;338:107–11.

14. Seldin DW, Rector FC, Jr. Symposium on acid–base homeostasis. The generation and maintenance of metabolic alkalosis. *Kidney Int* 1972;1:306–21.

15. Tuller MA, Mehdi F. Compensatory hypoventilation and hypercapnia in primary metabolic alkalosis. Report of three cases. *Am J Med* 1971;50:281–90.

16. Lifschitz MD, Brasch R, Cuomo AJ et al. Marked hypercapnia secondary to severe metabolic alkalosis. *Ann Intern Med* 1972;77:405–9.

17. Paulson WD. Effect of acute pH change on serum anion gap. *J Am Soc Nephrol* 1996;7:357–63.

18. Hood VL, Tannen RL. Protection of acid–base balance by pH regulation of acid production. *N Engl J Med* 1998;339:819–26.

19. Swartz RD, Rubin JE, Brown RS et al. Correction of postoperative metabolic alkalosis and renal failure by hemodialysis. *Ann Intern Med* 1977;86:52–5.

Part 2: Sodium and water balance

Richard N Hellman

Introduction

The nephrologist plays a critical role in fluid, electrolyte, and volume management in the intensive care unit (ICU) patient. The purpose of this chapter is to describe the functional management of these patients [1].

Volume control

Total body sodium, the major determinant of total body and extracellular fluid (ECF) volume, is regulated by sodium intake and renal sodium excretion. The serum sodium concentration relates to both total body sodium and total body water (TBW). TBW constitutes 45%–60% of total body weight, with two thirds in the intracellular fluid (ICF) compartment and one third in the ECF compartment. The ECF is divided into the interstitial and intravascular or plasma volume compartments. Fluid movement between the ECF and the ICF is driven by osmotic forces and cell membrane permeability, whereas fluid movement across capillary membranes between plasma and the interstitium is determined by hydrostatic and oncotic forces, and membrane permeability [2–5].

Renal sodium excretion is regulated by an afferent limb of volume sensors and an effector limb in the kidney – composed of the renin–angiotensin–aldosterone system, the glomerular filtration rate (GFR), physical factors, renal sympathetic nerves, and hormonal effective mechanisms such as vasopressin, catecholamines, prostaglandins, kinins, atrial natriuretic peptide, and endothelium-derived factors. Under physiologic conditions, urine sodium can increase in response to a sodium load or decrease in response to volume depletion [2–5].

The concept of effective arterial volume (EAV) is important in understanding the renal response to volume. The majority of total blood volume, 85%, is in the venous circulation, with only 15% in the arterial circulation. The EAV is the volume of blood in the arterial circulation that provides organ perfusion. Cardiac output and peripheral vascular resistance are the primary determinants of the arterial circulation. The ECF volume and the EAV can be independent of each other in edematous states – such as nephrotic syndrome, congestive heart failure (CHF), and cirrhosis – where the EAV is low despite edema and increased total body volume. **Table 1** compares total body volume and the EAV in various disease states, as well as the mechanism responsible for reduced EAV. Pathologic states of increased total body sodium with reduced renal sodium excretion are CHF, nephrotic syndrome, cirrhosis, hyperaldosteronism, and Liddle's syndrome. These entities will be discussed in **Section 2, Part 3** [2–5].

Table 1. A comparison of extracellular fluid volume, total blood volume, effective arterial volume, and pathophysiology in various disease states.

↑: increase; ↓: decrease; ↔: no change.

Pathologic state	Extracellular fluid volume	Total blood volume	Effective arterial volume	Pathophysiology
Congestive heart failure	↑	↑	↓	↓ Cardiac output
Cirrhosis (early)	↑	↑	↓	↓ Peripheral vascular resistance
Aortic stenosis	↑	↑	↓	Outlet obstruction
Sepsis	↔	↔	↓	↓ Peripheral vascular resistance
Nephrotic syndrome	↑	↓	↓	↓ Oncotic pressure
Gastrointestinal bleeding	↓	↓	↓	Vascular volume loss
Burn	↑	↓	↓	↓ Oncotic pressure ↑ Capillary leak

Water metabolism

Serum sodium concentration and osmolality are dependent on water metabolism. The major factors in water metabolism are thirst and antidiuretic hormone (ADH) or vasopressin. The major factors that affect thirst and ADH are listed in **Table 2**. Serum osmolality is maintained at a constant level, between 285 and 290 mOsm/L. Serum osmolality increases of 2%–3% stimulate thirst with a maximum osmotic threshold of 295 mOsm/kg of water. Vasopressin secretion is affected by plasma osmolality changes of 1%–2%, but volume stimulation outweighs osmolality changes if the blood volume is reduced by more than 7%. Nonosmotic vasopressin stimulation – eg, caused by pain, emesis, or morphine sulfate – is an important factor in postoperative hyponatremia [4,5].

The kidney's ability to concentrate and dilute the urine determines ECF osmolality and tonicity. ADH is the major factor controlling urine concentration and dilution in normal individuals. Under physiologic conditions, urine output can be as low as 500 mL/day or as high as 20–25 L/day. Urine may be concentrated, with an osmolality as high as 1,200 mOsm/kg, or dilute, with an osmolality of 50 mOsm/L. In the absence of ADH, or with fixed ADH secretion, urine output is dependent on solute (sodium, potassium salts, and urea) excretion. Free water is formed in the thick ascending limb of the loop of Henle and the ability to concentrate or dilute the urine is dependent on ADH [2–5].

Factors affecting free water formation are the GFR, proximal tubular reabsorption, the amount of filtrate delivered to the thick ascending limb, sodium chloride transport in the water-impermeable ascending limb of the loop of Henle, the length of the loop of Henle, medullary blood flow in the vasa recta, urea permeability in the collecting duct, and the cortical tubule responsiveness to ADH. If a low volume of glomerular filtration occurs, then less filtrate is delivered to the thick ascending limb of the loop of Henle and less free water

Table 2. Major factors affecting thirst and antidiuretic hormone (ADH).

ADH: antidiuretic hormone; P Osm: plasma osmolality; S Osm: serum osmolality.

Thirst	ADH vasopressin
Osmolality: S Osm Δ 2%–3% over basal levels, osmotic threshold of 295 mOsm/kg of water	Tonicity: P Osm Δ 1%–2%
Hypovolemia	Volume: effective arterial volume Δ>7%
Hypertension	Nonosmotic factors: eg, pain, emesis, hypoglycemia, angiotensin II, stress, exercise, fever, hypoxia, hypercapnia, morphine sulfate, and other drugs
ADH	
Angiotensin II	

is created. Patients with decreased creatinine clearances have reduced free water clearance. In a volume-depleted patient with hyponatremia, ADH levels are high and the ability to generate free water is lessened due to increased proximal tubular sodium reabsorption and reduced tubular fluid delivery to the thick ascending limb of the loop of Henle. Free water clearance quantifies the kidney's ability to concentrate and dilute the urine [2,3].

Clinical assessment of volume in the patient

The nephrologist's approach to the ICU patient always involves taking a careful history and performing a physical examination (PE), focusing on volume assessment, hemodynamics, fluid balance, weight, urine output, and medications being taken. A history of volume loss – such as vomiting, diarrhea, nasogastric suction, gastrointestinal bleeding, "third space" losses, or excessive diuresis – may be present. In the ICU setting, postoperative fluid gains or losses and total parenteral nutrition (TPN) administration need to be identified and quantified. Indications of volume depletion include decreased weight, intake<output, orthostatic hypotension, dry mucus membranes, skin tenting, an elevated blood urea nitrogen to creatinine ratio (BUN:Cr), and a reduced fractional excretion of sodium (FENa), central venous pressure, or pulmonary capillary wedge pressure [6].

Hyponatremia

Definition

Hyponatremia is defined as a serum sodium concentration of <135 mmol/L. Clinically significant hyponatremia is usually defined as serum sodium of <130 mmol/L, and symptomatic hyponatremia usually occurs when serum sodium goes below 120 mmol/L. Severe hyponatremia is defined as serum sodium of <115 mmol/L. The symptoms and signs of hyponatremia primarily relate to the central nervous system (CNS) (see **Table 3**) [1–5,7–9].

Pseudohyponatremia is a methodologic artifactual reduction in serum sodium due to displacement of a portion of the water phase of plasma by lipid or protein. It is observed by flame emission spectrometry measurement, but can be avoided with use of a sodium selective electrode without dilution. Pseudohyponatremia needs to be excluded as a cause of false hyponatremia. Hyperlipidemia and hyperproteinemia, as occurs in multiple myeloma,

Table 3. Symptoms and signs of hyponatremia.

[a]Symptom of hyponatremia with small cell carcinoma of the lung.

Symptoms	Signs
Lethargy	Abnormal sensorium
Apathy	Depressed deep tendon reflexes
Disorientation	Cheyne–Stokes respiration
Muscle cramps	Hypothermia
Anorexia	Pathologic reflexes
Nausea	Pseudobulbar palsy
Agitation	Seizures
Dysgeusia (sweet taste)[a]	

can cause pseudohyponatremia. In true hyponatremia, effective osmolality is low but total body sodium and TBW levels may be decreased, normal, or increased. In pseudohyponatremia, these variables are unchanged from normal [10].

Relationship between serum sodium and serum osmolality

Serum sodium is the major determinant of serum osmolality (S Osm). The normal measured S Osm is 285–290 mOsm/L [2–5]. The S Osm can be calculated using the following formula:

$$\text{S Osm} = (2)[\text{serum sodium}] + \text{BUN}/2.8 + [\text{glucose}]/18$$

Calculation of the S Osm is a useful measurement in patients with hyponatremia and metabolic acidosis. The difference between the measured and calculated osmolality yields the osmolar gap. A value of <10 mOsm/L is normal for the osmolar gap. The effective osmolality or tonicity is the part of total osmolality that has the potential to cause transmembrane water movement between the ECF and ICF compartments. Effective solutes – such as sodium or mannitol – are confined to the ECF. Ineffective solutes – such as urea and ethanol – freely pass between the ECF and the ICF. There is a risk of developing cerebral edema if the ECF osmolality is less than the ICF osmolality, favoring water movement from the hypotonic ECF to the hypertonic ICF. Therefore, hyponatremia is a major concern in the development of cerebral edema [10].

Translocational hyponatremia represents a shift of water from the ICF to the ECF space, not an increase in TBW. Glucose, mannitol, glycine, maltose, glycerol, sorbitol, and radio contrast agents increase serum osmolality and decrease serum sodium concentrations, causing translocational hyponatremia, whereas membrane-permeant solutes – such as urea, ethanol, ethylene glycol, isopropyl alcohol, and methanol – increase serum osmolality but have no effect on serum sodium (see **Table 4**) [10].

Correction factors for hyperglycemia

Hyperglycemia accounts for 16% of hyponatremia cases [7]. As hyponatremia is translocational, correction factors are necessary for hyponatremia in hyperglycemia cases. The Katz correction factor for hyperglycemia estimates a 1.6 mEq/L fall in serum sodium for each 100 mg/dL increase in serum glucose. The Hillier correction calls for a fall in serum sodium of 2.4 mEq/L for each increase in serum glucose of 100 mg/dL, and it appears to be more accurate if blood glucose is >400 mg/dL [11,12].

Table 4. Typical pitfalls in the diagnosis of hyponatremia.

S Na^+: serum sodium; S Osm: serum osmolality.

Normal S Osm/normal S Na^+ (pseudohyponatremia)	Increased S Osm/ decreased S Na^+	Increased S Osm/ normal S Na^+
Hyperlipidemia	Glucose	Urea
Hyperproteinemia	Mannitol	Ethanol
	Glycine	Ethylene glycol
	Maltose	Isopropylalcohol
	Glycerol	Methanol
	Sorbitol	
	Radio contrast agents	

Demographics

Hyponatremia is the most common electrolyte abnormality seen in the general hospital patient. Hyponatremia is a marker for underlying severe disease, and the degree of hyponatremia correlates with the severity of CHF. It is hospital acquired in two thirds of patients, which is why it is important in the ICU setting. Prevention of hyponatremia is key to good management, just as it is in other fluid, electrolyte, and acid–base problems. Hyponatremia has a daily incidence of 0.97% and a prevalence of 2.5%. It is seen postoperatively in 4.4% of patients. Patients with hyponatremia have a 60-times higher fatality rate than those with normonatremia. The majority of hospitalized patients with hyponatremia (97%) have nonosmotic vasopressin secretion [2,3,5,7].

Signs and symptoms of hyponatremia

The signs and symptoms of hyponatremia are related to the CNS and are listed in **Table 3**. Brain adaptation to hyponatremia involves the loss of sodium, potassium, and organic osmols to prevent the development of cerebral edema. This brain compensation occurs over a 48-hour period. Therefore, rapid correction of hyponatremia may result in brain shrinkage and the development of osmotic demyelination syndrome (ODS).

Mechanisms of hyponatremia can consist of pure water excess, pure solute loss, and mixed abnormalities [1]. Hyponatremia can occur with hypervolemia – such as in CHF, renal failure, nephrotic syndrome, and hepatic cirrhosis – as hypovolemic hyponatremia related to renal or extrarenal losses, or as euvolemic hyponatremia (see **Table 5**). The causes of hyponatremia are listed in **Table 6** [1–3].

Diagnosis of hyponatremia

Pertinent assessment of the hyponatremic patient includes taking a careful history and PE, including a complete drug history. The PE should assess the volume status of the patient, looking for the presence or absence of edema, or signs of CHF, liver disease, or kidney disease. Laboratory analysis should include tests for BUN, creatinine, electrolytes, calcium, phosphorous, albumen, serum osmolality, and spot urine tests for Na^+, K^+, Cl^-, and creatinine. Specialized laboratory testing should be ordered according to the potential causes in the individual patient. These tests should include thyroid-stimulating hormone,

Table 5. Clinical circumstances associated with hyponatremia in the intensive care unit (ICU) patient.

SIADH: syndrome of inappropriate antidiuretic hormone secretion.
Reproduced with permission from Berl T, Anderson RJ, McDonald KM et al. Clinical disorders of water metabolism. *Kidney Int* 1976;10:117–32.

ICU clinical circumstances associated with hyponatremia
Pseudohyponatremia
Hypervolemia hyponatremia
- Congestive heart failure
- Chronic kidney disease/acute renal failure
- Nephrotic syndrome
- Hepatic cirrhosis
Hypovolemic hyponatremia
Euvolemic hyponatremia
- SIADH
- Endocrine disorders, eg, Addison's disease, hypothyroidism
- Pharmacologic agents
- Emotional and physical stress

serum cortisol, and Cortrosyn stimulation tests, liver function tests, a tuberculosis skin test, and a porphyrin screen in patients with unexplained syndrome of inappropriate antidiuretic hormone secretion (SIADH). Initial volume assessment is critical, with patients being categorized as hypovolemic, hypervolemic, or euvolemic. A systematic approach for the diagnosis of hyponatremia is provided in **Figure 1** [1–3].

Hypovolemic hyponatremia

In hypovolemic hyponatremia, total body sodium is reduced to a greater extent than TBW, resulting in hyponatremia. Renal losses are most likely in cases where the urine sodium is >20 mmol/L. Extrarenal losses are most likely if the urine sodium is <20 mmol/L [2,3]. Clinical prediction of hypovolemia in hyponatremia often lacks sensitivity despite good specificity. The combination of a low FENa (<0.5%) and a low fractional excretion of urea (<2%) is the best way to predict a response to saline. The presence of a high fractional excretion of potassium in this situation suggests diuretic intake. Elevated BUN:Cr ratio, serum uric acid, hematocrit, and serum protein concentrations are suggestive of volume depletion [6].

Hypervolemic hyponatremia

Hypervolemic hyponatremia is associated with an increase in total body sodium and a greater increase in TBW. If urine sodium is >20 mmol/L in the absence of diuretics, acute or chronic renal failure is likely. If the urine sodium is <20 mmol/L, nephrotic syndrome, cirrhosis, or CHF are the most likely diagnoses. In these disease processes, a reduced EAV results in sodium retention and nonosmotic stimulation of ADH secretion.

Euvolemic hyponatremia

Euvolemic hyponatremia is associated with normal total body sodium and an increase in TBW. It is the most common form of hyponatremia observed in hospitalized patients. The urine sodium is >20 mmol/L in these patients. The differential diagnosis of this type of hyponatremia includes glucocorticoid deficiency, hypothyroidism, stress, medications, and SIADH.

Table 6. Causes of hypotonic hyponatremia.

Reproduced with permission from Adrogué HJ, Madias NE. Hyponatremia. *N Engl J Med* 2000;342:1581–9.

Hypovolemic	
Renal sodium loss	**Extrarenal sodium loss**
Diuretic agents	Diarrhea
Osmotic diuresis (glucose, urea, mannitol)	Vomiting
Adrenal insufficiency	Blood loss
Salt-wasting nephropathy	Excessive sweating (eg, in marathon runners)
Cerebral salt wasting	Fluid sequestration in "third space"
Bicarbonaturia (renal tubular acidosis, disequilibrium stage of vomiting)	
Ketonuria	
Hypervolemic	
Congenital heart failure	
Cirrhosis	
Nephrotic syndrome	
Renal failure (acute or chronic)	
Pregnancy	
Euvolemic	
Thiazide diuretics	Pulmonary conditions – Infections – Acute respiratory failure – Positive-pressure ventilation
Hypothyroidism	Miscellaneous – Postoperative state – Pain – Severe nausea – Infection with the human immunodeficiency virus – Porphyria (acute intermittent porphyria)
Adrenal insufficiency	Decreased intake of solutes – Beer potomania – Tea and toast diet
Syndrome of inappropriate secretion of antidiuretic hormone	Excessive water intake – Primary polydipsia – Dilute infant formula – Sodium-free solutions (used in hysteroscopy, laparoscopy, or transurethral resection of the prostate) – Accidental intake of large amounts of water – Multiple tap-water enemas
Cancer – Pulmonary tumors – Mediastinal tumors – Extrathoracic tumors	
Central nervous system disorders – Acute psychosis – Mass lesions – Inflammatory and demyelinating diseases – Stroke – Hemorrhage – Trauma	
Drugs – Desmopressin – Oxytocin – Prostaglandin-synthesis inhibitors – Nicotine – Phenothiazines – Tricyclic antidepressants – Serotonin-reuptake inhibitors – Opiate derivatives – Chlorpropamide – Clofibrate – Carbamazepine – Cyclophosphamide – Vincristine	

Figure 1. Diagnostic approach to the hyponatremia patient.

SIADH: syndrome of inappropriate antidiuretic hormone secretion; U Na: urinary sodium.
Reprinted from *Comprehensive Clinical Nephrology*, Johnson JR, Feehally J, editors. Chapter 9: Disorders of water metabolism, Berl T, Kumar S:9.1–9.20. Copyright 2004, with permission from Elsevier.

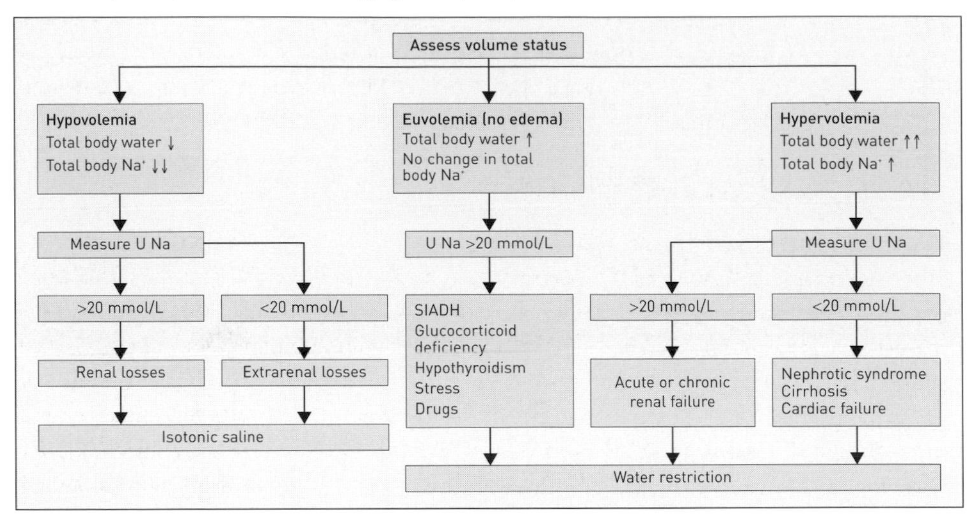

Figure 2. Treatment of severe euvolemic hyponatremia (serum sodium [S Na⁺] <115–120 mmol/L).
CT: computed tomography; MRI: magnetic resonance imaging.
[a]Consider mannitol if hypertonic saline not available.
Reprinted from *Comprehensive Clinical Nephrology*, Johnson JR, Feehally J, editors. Chapter 9: Disorders of water metabolism, Berl T, Kumar S:9.1–9.20. Copyright 2004, with permission from Elsevier.

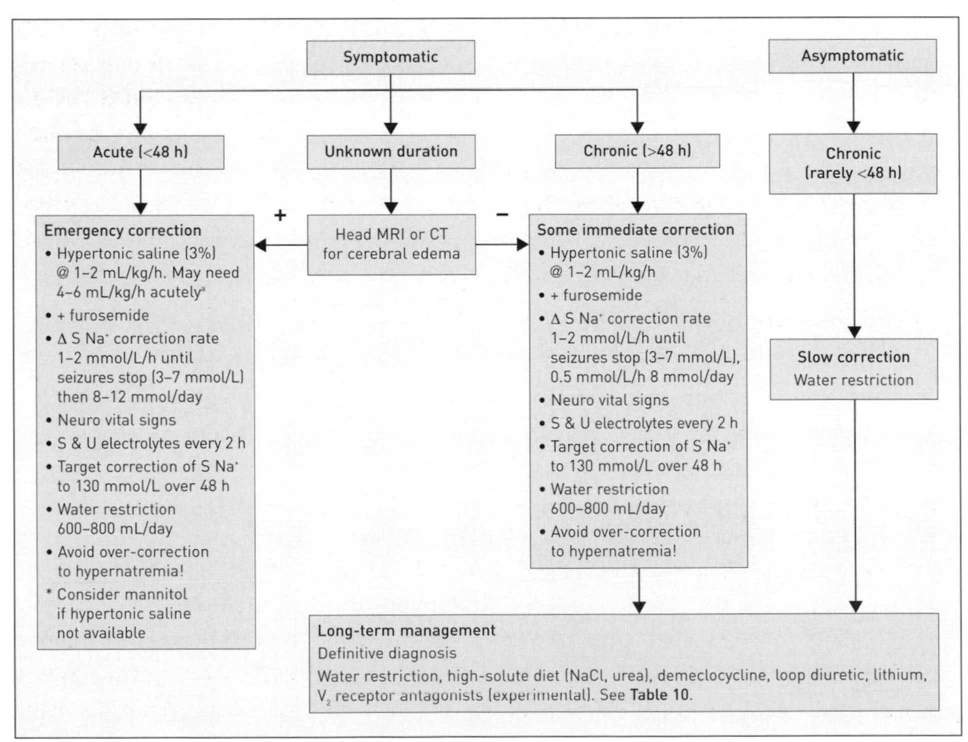

Syndrome of inappropriate antidiuretic hormone secretion

The diagnostic criteria for SIADH are hyponatremia and hypo-osmolality, urine that is less than maximally dilute, urine sodium matching intake despite hyponatremia, nonsuppressible plasma ADH, no evidence of cardiac, hepatic, renal, adrenal, thyroid, or pituitary disease, and improvement of renal sodium wasting and hyponatremia with rigid water restriction. Water restriction improves hyponatremia caused by SIADH. Hypouricemia is commonly observed with SIADH because of increased renal uric acid secretion [13].

Treatment of hyponatremia

The general approach to the diagnosis and treatment of the hyponatremic patient is described in **Figure 1**. A serum sodium of <130 mmol/L should be the trigger for initiation of treatment. The cause of the hyponatremia should be ascertained, addressed, and water restriction begun, if appropriate, with slow correction. Symptomatic hyponatremia in patients with serum sodium of <120–125 mmol/L generally needs more aggressive management. Treatment of Addison's disease with glucocorticoids and mineralocorticoids, and treatment of hypothyroidism, are obviously important in the management of these hyponatremias. Glucocorticoids and mineralocorticoids may have a role in the critically ill ICU patient with hypothalamic–pituitary–adrenal dysfunction [1–3,14].

Hypovolemic hyponatremia

Treatment of hypovolemic hyponatremia involves discontinuation of any offending agents – such as diuretics – followed by administration of isotonic saline and potassium repletion. Volume repletion allows increased delivery of filtrate to the thick ascending limb of the loop of Henle and increased free water production. It also suppresses volume-regulated ADH. Urinary dilution can then take place with increased free water excretion. The importance of the rate of correction in this circumstance in terms of ODS is uncertain. ODS has been described with all forms of hyponatremia, and the chronicity of hyponatremia may be an important factor. Slower correction of chronic hypovolemic hyponatremia would seem prudent. Careful monitoring of the neurologic status, volume status, and electrolytes is indicated until hyponatremia is corrected. Hypertonic saline is usually unnecessary in this situation, but can be used in patients with severe symptomatic hyponatremia [1–3,5].

Hypervolemic hyponatremia

Hypervolemic hyponatremia is treated with sodium and water restriction and diuretics. In cirrhosis, the diuretic spironolactone is the first to be utilized with subsequent use of thiazide or loop diuretics if there is inadequate diuresis. Hypertonic saline is contraindicated as the patient already has increased total body sodium [2,3,5].

Euvolemic hyponatremia

Symptomatic – acute and chronic

Acute symptomatic hyponatremia is a medical emergency and nephrologists agree that it needs more rapid correction because of the risk of cerebral edema. In those cases where the duration of hyponatremia is unknown, a computed tomography (CT) or magnetic resonance image (MRI) of the head, specifically looking for cerebral edema, may be helpful.

Table 7. Acute neurologic syndromes associated with osmotic demyelination syndrome (ODS).

Acute neurologic syndrome	Clinical characteristics
Altered mental status	Occurs 1–11 days post hyponatremia correction
Flaccid quadraparesis	Poor prognosis
Dysconjugate eye movement	Reintroduction of hyponatremia after overshoot hypernatremia may prevent ODS
Pseudobulbar palsy	
Pontine localization	
Edema	
Demyelination of gray and white matter	

Table 8. A typical example showing the calculation of the desired negative water balance. Total body water (TBW) in liters as a percentage of body weight in kilograms is estimated at 60% in children and men, 50% in women and elderly men, and 45% in elderly women.

SIADH: syndrome of inappropriate antidiuretic hormone secretion; S Na^+: serum sodium concentration.

Calculation of desired negative water balance
A 40-year-old, euvolemic, 70-kg male with SIADH, seizures, normokalemia, and S Na^+ of 113 mEq/L
TBW = (70) × (0.6) = 42 L
$\left(\frac{\text{Actual S Na}^+}{\text{Desired S Na}^+}\right) \times (\text{TBW}) = \left(\frac{113}{130}\right) \times (42) = 36.5\text{ L}$
TBW (excess) for an S Na^+ of 130 mEq/L = 42 – 36.5 = 5.5 L negative water balance to increase plasma Na^+ from 113 mEq/L to 130 mEq/L

Symptomatic hyponatremia is usual when the serum sodium level is <115–120 mmol/L (see **Figure 2**) [1–5,8,9].

Groups at risk for symptomatic hyponatremia are menstruating women, elderly women on thiazides, children, hypoxic patients, and patients with psychogenic polydipsia. In symptomatic acute hyponatremia of <48 hours duration, more rapid correction, initially 1–2 mmol/h but not exceeding 8–10 mmol/day, may be necessary. Even in patients with seizures and hyponatremia, a small correction of 1–6 mmol is usually associated with resolution of neurologic symptoms.

Osmotic demyelination syndrome

Euvolemic hyponatremia due to SIADH poses a particular management problem. These cases often present with hyponatremia of chronicity, and, as such, are more likely to be adversely affected by overly rapid correction. ODS, possibly developing as a result of rapid correction of hyponatremia, has been a particularly devastating complication of therapy. High-risk groups for ODS are alcoholics, malnourished patients, hypokalemic patients, burn patients, patients with liver disease, and elderly women on thiazide diuretics. The clinical characteristics and factors predisposing to ODS are listed in **Table 7**. The diagnosis of ODS is made using MRI, which may not be positive until 2 weeks after symptoms occur. The usual clinical presentation is the development of neurologic symptoms 2–3 days after correction of hyponatremia. To minimize the risk of ODS, a rate of correction of no more than 8–10 mmol/day has been recommended for all hyponatremic patients [1–5,8,9].

Table 9a. Clinically useful formulae for estimating the effect of 1 L of infusate (I) on the serum sodium level (S Na^+). These equations assume a pure water excess and do not account for ongoing solute (Na^+ or K^+) loss or gain.

Δ S Na^+: change in serum sodium level per liter of infusate; TBW: total body water.

Reproduced with permission from Adrogué HJ, Madias NE. Hyponatremia. *N Engl J Med* 2000;342:1581–9.

Formula	Clinical use
(a) $\Delta S\,Na^+ = \dfrac{I\,Na^+ - S\,Na^+}{TBW + 1}$	Estimated effect of 1 L of infusate on S Na^+
(b) $\Delta S\,Na^+ = \dfrac{(I\,Na^+ + I\,K^+) - (S\,Na^+)}{TBW + 1}$	

Table 9b. Infusates used in the clinical treatment of hyponatremia.

Reproduced with permission from Adrogué HJ, Madias NE. Hyponatremia. *N Engl J Med* 2000;342:1581–9.

Infusate intravenous fluid	Infusate sodium (mmol/L)	Extracellular fluid distribution (%)
3% NaCl in water	513	100
0.9% NaCl in water	154	100
Ringer lactate solution	130	97
0.45% NaCl in water	77	73
0.2% NaCl in 5% dextrose in water	34	55
5% Dextrose in water	0	40

Calculation of the desired negative water balance

Definitive treatment of hyponatremia begins with calculation of the desired negative water balance (see **Table 8**). Adrogué and Madias have provided a clinically useful way of estimating the effect of 1 L of infusate on serum sodium (formula b should be used if potassium is added to the infusate) (see **Tables 9a** and **9b**).

Limitations of this method include the assumption of a pure water excess, lack of consideration of ongoing solute loss, and insensible loss. An advantage is the automatic linkage of therapy with water balance. However, formulae for correction of hyponatremia provide guidelines for management. The rate of correction in the patient must be monitored regularly to determine the appropriate rate of correction and to avoid over-correction to hypernatremia [1].

An initial infusion rate for 3% NaCl can be estimated by the product of the desired rate of increase in serum sodium (mEq/L/h) and the patient's weight in kilograms. A 70 kg patient with acute symptomatic hyponatremia in whom a rate of serum sodium increase of 1 mEq/L is required will need 3% NaCl at 70 mL/h. If the desired rate of correction is 0.5 mEq/h, then the infusion rate for 3% NaCl is 35 mL/h [2].

Loop diuretics, like furosemide, produce large volumes of hypotonic urine (urinary sodium approximately 75 mEq/L). This, combined with infusion of hypertonic saline (3% saline), or even isotonic saline (0.9%), will hasten the correction of hyponatremia.

Table 10. Treatment of chronic asymptomatic hyponatremia.
Reprinted from *Comprehensive Clinical Nephrology*, Johnson JR, Feehally J, editors. Chapter 9: Disorders of water metabolism, Berl T, Kumar S:9.1–9.20. Copyright 2004, with permission from Elsevier.

Treatment	Mechanism of action	Dose	Advantages	Limitations
Fluid restriction	Decreases availability of free water	Variable	Effective and inexpensive Not complicated	Noncompliance
Pharmacologic inhibition of vasopressin action				
Lithium	Inhibits the kidney's response to vasopressin	900–1,200 mg daily	Unrestricted water intake	Polyuria, narrow therapeutic range, neurotoxicity
Demeclocycline	Inhibits the kidney's response to vasopressin	300–600 mg twice daily	Effective; unrestricted water intake	Neurotoxcicity, polyuria, photosensitivity, nephrotoxicity. Allow 2 weeks for effect
V_2 receptor antagonist	Antagonizes vasopressin action	–	–	–
Increased solute intake				
Furosemide (frusemide)	Increases free water clearance	Titrate to optimal dose; coadministration of 2–3 g NaCl	Effective	Ototoxicity, K^+ depletion
Urea	Osmotic diuresis	30–60 g daily	Effective; unrestricted water intake; immediate effect	Polyuria, unpalatable, gastrointestinal symptoms

Serum sodium will increase as long as the infusate concentration of sodium plus potassium exceeds the concentration of urinary sodium and potassium. The goal is to keep the amount of sodium infused and the urinary sodium equal. In this way, the volume status of the patient does not change (total body sodium), but free water is lost in the urine [1–3].

The patient described in **Table 8** is treated with 3% saline (**Table 9b**) at a rate of 70 mL/h for 7 hours (490 mL). After 2 hours he is awake and alert and has no further seizures. Intravenous furosemide was given.

$$\Delta \text{ S Na}^+ = \frac{\text{I Na}^+ - \text{S Na}^+}{\text{TBW} + 1} = \frac{513 - 113}{43} = 9.3 \text{ mEq/L}$$

One half liter of 3% saline would be expected to increase the serum sodium level by 4.65 or 5 mEq/L to 118 mEq/L in the absence of ongoing sodium loss. The serum sodium level is 120 mEq/L after 7 hours. The target rate of correction is 8–10 mEq/day.

The correction of hyponatremia should include careful monitoring of the neurologic status, vital signs, and fluid balance. It is prudent to check serum and urinary electrolytes every 2 hours for the first 24 hours and then every 4–6 hours until hyponatremia is corrected to 130 mEq/L. While hypertonic saline is necessary in symptomatic hyponatremia, the high sodium content cannot be forgotten. Limiting use to the initial correction and paying attention to signs of volume overload are necessary. Using >500 mL of 3% saline is usually not necessary. Aggressive acute correction of hyponatremia can cease when symptoms have resolved and serum sodium is >120–125 mmol/L. At this point, water restriction alone and implementation of strategies listed for the therapy of chronic asymptomatic hyponatremia can be initiated (see **Table 10**).

Over-correction of hyponatremia is absolutely contraindicated. If over-correction of hyponatremia to overt hypernatremia occurs with CNS symptoms, animal data suggest that the return to moderate hyponatremia may be effective in preventing ODS [9,15].

Chronic asymptomatic hyponatremia

Most experts stress a conservative approach to treatment of asymptomatic hyponatremia with water restriction despite severity. Chronic hyponatremia management in SIADH patients has included a high-salt diet, urea, furosemide, lithium, demeclocycline, and phenytoin sodium. Treatment of chronic asymptomatic hyponatremia therapy is summarized in **Table 10**. V_2 receptor antagonists (aquaretics) are a new class of drug that inhibit vasopressin binding. They inhibit the action of vasopressin by blocking the V_2 receptor and are a promising experimental therapy for chronic euvolemic and hypervolemic hyponatremia.

In summary, hyponatremia is a common problem in the hospitalized patient. Clinical history, assessment of volume status, exclusion of pseudohyponatremia and translocational hyponatremia, and urine sodium measurement assist in the diagnosis and rational treatment. Acute symptomatic severe hyponatremia, with attendant cerebral edema, is a medical emergency requiring prompt recognition and treatment with hypertonic saline and furosemide. Minimal corrections of serum sodium usually promptly resolve CNS symptoms. Slow correction of hyponatremia, with target rates of 8–10 mmol/day, is recommended in all patients to avoid ODS. CT and MRI scanning of the brain may be helpful when the duration of hyponatremia is uncertain. Appropriate clinical monitoring and avoidance of hypotonic fluids in postoperative patients and those at high risk for hyponatremia can lead to successful prevention and minimization of severe hyponatremia in the hospitalized, critically ill patient.

Hypernatremia

Introduction

Hypernatremia is a common problem in the ICU. It is always associated with hyperosmolality and some degree of cellular dehydration. Major signs and symptoms of hypernatremia are related to the CNS [16].

Definition

Hypernatremia is defined as a serum sodium level of >145 mEq/L [2,16,17]. Symptoms usually appear if serum sodium is >160 mEq/L; however, a 36% mortality was noted in one study in which the peak serum sodium was 149 mEq/L [18]. Survival has been described if serum sodium is >200 mEq/L, but this is rare [19].

Figure 3. Differential diagnosis of the hypernatremia patient.
Reproduced with permission from Berl T, Anderson RJ, McDonald KM et al. Clinical disorders of water metabolism. *Kidney Int* 1976;10:117–32.

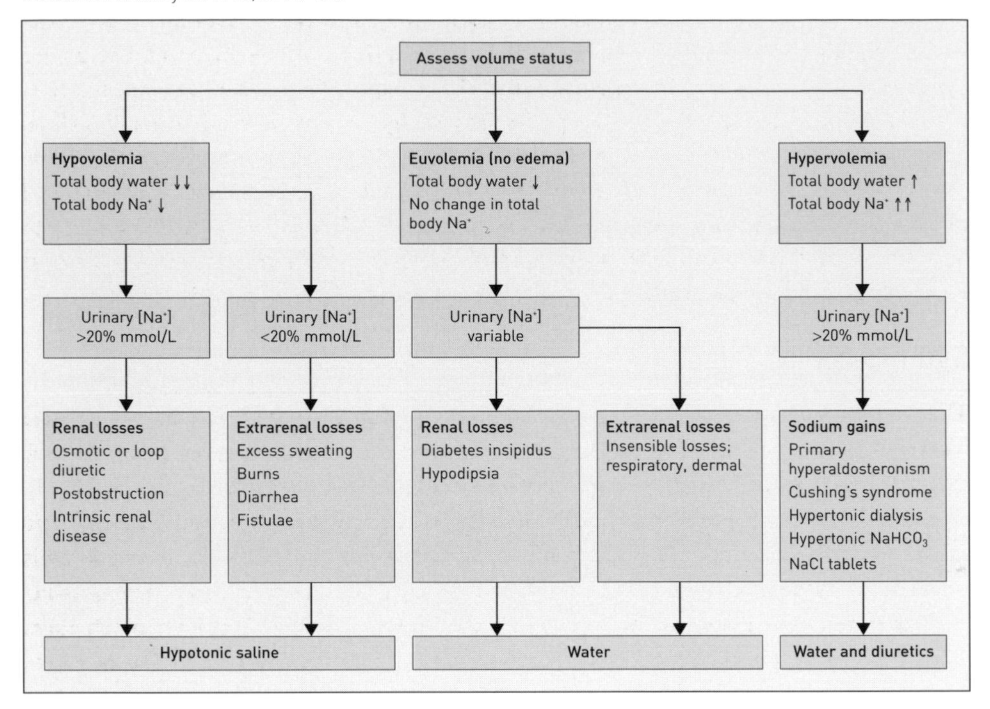

Demographics

The incidence of hypernatremia in the hospital has been reported to be between 0.7% and 4.1%, with a mortality ranging between 42% and 60%. Morbidity is high and 10%–15% of children have a neurologic deficit post-treatment for hypernatremia. Hypernatremia is hospital acquired 57% of the time and this form has a higher mortality than hypernatremia diagnosed at hospital admission [18,20]. Hypernatremia that develops in hospital is often associated with edema and hypervolemia related to large volumes of isotonic fluid, and is associated with a mortality of 32% [21]. In one series, hypernatremia present on admission was associated with hypovolemia, had a mortality rate of 20%, and was rapidly corrected, whereas hypernatremia that developed in hospital had no or inadequate correction and was associated with a mortality rate of 32% [20].

Predisposing factors and prevention

Hypernatremia is a disease that occurs at the extremes of age. Inadequate amounts of free water intake, hypodipsic syndromes, increased insensible losses, CNS disease, infirmity, and lack of water access with hypotonic fluid loss predispose to hypernatremia [16]. In one series, the most frequent causes of hypernatremia were complications of surgery, febrile illness, infirmity, and diabetes mellitus. In patients with diabetes insipidus – central or nephrogenic – normal thirst allows the maintenance of normonatremia. When these patients are denied access to water, such as postoperatively, large urinary free water losses can occur, leading to hypernatremia. Therefore, prevention of hypernatremia is perhaps the most important thing to do for the patient. ICU patients with altered sensorium, mechanical ventilation, managed access to water, and those receiving large volumes of isotonic or hypertonic fluid are at risk for hypernatremia. This is especially true for patients on a loop diuretic. Loop diuretics obligate the production of hypo-osmotic urine (urinary sodium approximately 75 mEq/L), and, if intravenous replacement fluids are of greater osmolality, serum sodium will increase. Anticipation of free water needs in patients on loop diuretics and in patients with increased insensible loss, assurance of adequate free water intake with intravenous TPN and tube feedings, and control of blood glucose to avoid osmotic diuresis are all steps that need to be taken to protect the patient from hypernatremia [22].

Symptoms

The symptoms of hypernatremia include initial intense thirst, altered consciousness, muscle weakness, seizures, and coma. In children, hyperpnea, muscle weakness, restlessness, insomnia, lethargy, and a high-pitched cry may be present. Seizures and coma also occur [16]. Hypernatremia can lead to brain shrinkage with vascular rupture, cerebral bleeding, and subarachnoid hemorrhage. The depression of sensorium in a patient with hypernatremia correlates with the level of serum sodium [16,18,23]. CNS adaptation includes accumulation of electrolytes with restoration of brain water and volume [16,24]. Therefore, overly rapid correction of long-standing hypernatremia can produce cerebral edema in the hyperosmolar brain, leading to coma, convulsions, and death. This is why correction of hypernatremia needs to be done gradually [16].

Mechanisms of hypernatremia

Hypernatremia occurs as a result of pure water loss, pure solute gain, water shifts from the ECF to the ICF, and mixed conditions. Pure water loss may be due to defects in urine concentrating mechanisms such as in diabetes insipidus, water loss due to insensible loss from fever, or inadequate water intake. Pure solute gain occurs in the presence of salt poisoning. Water shifts from the ECF to the ICF can occur with seizures and exercise [2,16,17,25,26]. Net water loss accounts for the majority of cases of hypernatremia.

Causes and differential diagnosis of hypernatremia

The causes and differential diagnosis of hypernatremia can be categorized on the basis of their mechanisms (see **Figure 3**). Net water loss can be due to hypotonic fluid loss or pure water loss. These losses may be renal or extrarenal. The loss of hypotonic fluid is usually associated with hypovolemia and is termed hypovolemic hypernatremia. Pure water loss is usually observed along with normal total body sodium and is termed euvolemic hyponatremia. Hypertonic sodium gain is called hypervolemic hypernatremia [2,25].

Hypovolemic hypernatremia is due to either renal or extrarenal loss of hypotonic fluids. TBW is decreased to a greater extent than the total body sodium. If urine sodium is high, renal losses are indicated; if urine sodium is low, extrarenal losses are indicated [2].

Figure 4. Management of hypernatremia.

DI: diabetes insipidus; DM: diabetes mellitus; S Na^+: serum sodium level; SQ: subcutaneously.

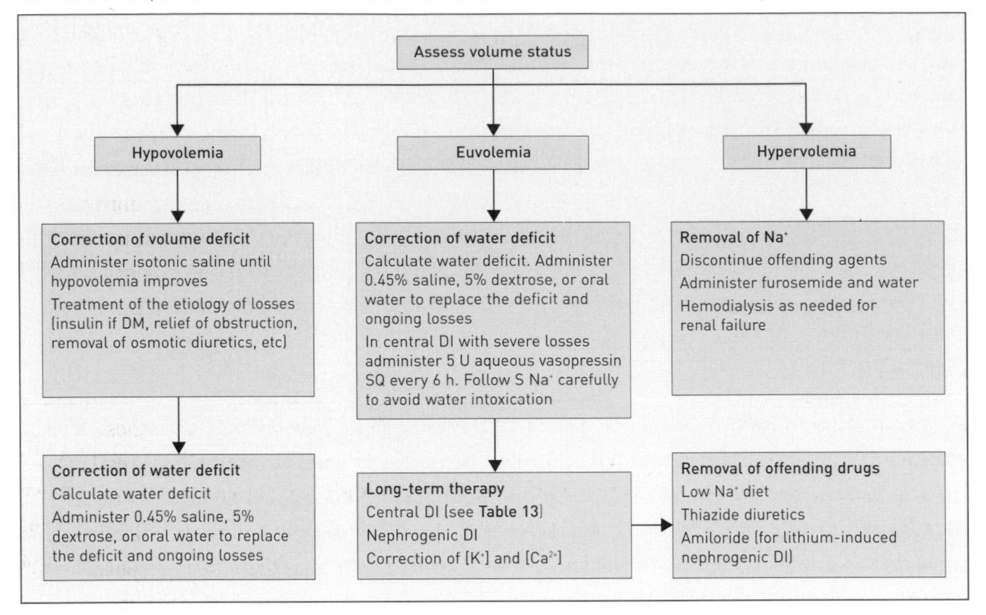

Hypervolemic hypernatremia is associated with edema and a total body sodium increase greater than the TBW increase. Urine sodium tends to be high [2].

Euvolemic hypernatremia is associated with no edema, no change in total body sodium, and a decrease in TBW. Urine sodium is variable [2].

In the ICU, central (neurogenic) diabetes insipidus can be either acquired or congenital, leading to euvolemic hypernatremia. In either case there is a deficiency of ADH due to reduced production and/or secretion. ADH works on the kidney at the level of the cortical collecting duct (CCD) by binding to a basolateral V_2 receptor. This interaction increases production of cyclic AMP and apical aquaporin-2 (AQP2) insertion [2,25], leading to increased CCD water permeability and, consequently, enhanced water reabsorption. Causes of acquired central diabetes insipidus are post-traumatic, postsurgical, tumors, histiocytosis, granulomas – such as sarcoidosis and tuberculosis – aneurysm, meningitis, encephalitis, Guillain–Barré syndrome, and idiopathic [2,25].

Net pure water loss can also occur with nephrogenic diabetes insipidus, which is either a rare congenital form of the condition or is acquired [2,25,27,28]. Chronic kidney disease, hypokalemia, protein malnutrition, and lithium therapy all lead to downregulation of AQP2 and a reduced reabsorptive capacity for water. Therefore, acquired nephrogenic diabetes insipidus can occur with hypokalemia, hypercalcemia, chronic kidney disease, the diuretic phase of acute tubular necrosis, postobstructive diuresis, and protein malnutrition. Medications such as demeclocycline, lithium, foscarnet, or amphotericin B, as well as pregnancy, which can be associated with placental secretion of vasopressinase, can cause acquired nephrogenic diabetes insipidus [2,29].

Table 11. Hypernatremia: general principles of treatment.

Address the underlying cause
Control fever
Minimize gastrointestinal or renal losses
Control blood glucose
Correct hypercalcemia
Correct hypokalemia
Increase free water in nasogastric tube feedings
Hypotonic fluid replacement
Use oral or enteral water if possible
Slow correction
Isotonic saline (0.9% NaCl) to be used only if there is circulatory compromise
Calculate the water deficit

A typical presentation in the ICU would be a neurosurgical patient with acute onset of polyuria and central diabetes insipidus post head trauma. Polyuria (urine output >3–4 L/day) is the common feature of diabetes insipidus. The differential diagnosis of polyuria includes partial and complete central or nephrogenic diabetes insipidus, primary polyuria, intrinsic renal disease, and osmotic diuresis. Hypernatremia in diabetes insipidus occurs if the patient cannot exercise the normal thirst mechanism.

The water deprivation test can be used to differentiate the causes of polyuria. Primary polyuria is associated with normal or hyponatremia [2]. The kidney responds to water deprivation and vasopressin in central complete or partial diabetes insipidus with an increase in urine osmolality. There is no response with nephrogenic diabetes insipidus. In the acutely ill patient with polyuria in the ICU, the water deprivation test is often not feasible and a test dose of vasopressin is usually given after causes of nephrogenic diabetes insipidus have been ruled out.

Treatment of hypernatremia

General measures in the treatment of hypernatremia are the identification of underlying causes; the duration, severity, symptoms, and type of hypernatremia; and calculation of the water deficit (see **Figure 4** and **Table 11**) [2,16]. The following formula can be used to calculate the water deficit:

$$\mathbf{0.4 \times (lean\ body\ weight\ in\ kg) \times \left[\frac{(serum\ Na^{+})}{140} - 1\right]}$$

This formula assumes that TBW in liters is 40% of total lean body weight in kilograms for adult men and women irrespective of age, and calculates the water deficit necessary to correct serum sodium to 140 mEq/L.

In acute symptomatic hypernatremia of several hours' duration, more rapid correction at rates of 1 mEq/L/h initially until symptoms resolve, followed by 8–10 mEq/L/day, are appropriate, as brain hyperosmolality has not yet developed. Once symptoms have resolved, the remainder of the water deficit can be replaced over 24–48 hours [17]. The target serum sodium level is 140–145 mEq/L [16]. Neurological vital signs, intake and output, daily weight,

Table 12. Characteristics of infusates used to treat hypernatremia.
D5: 5% dextrose.
Reproduced with permission from Adrogué HJ, Madias NE. Hypernatremia. *N Engl J Med* 2000;342:1493–9.

Infusate	Infusate sodium (mmol/L)	Extracellular fluid distribution
D5 in water	0	40
D5 0.2% NaCl	34	55
D5 0.45% NaCl	77	73
Ringer's lactate	130	97
0.9% NaCl	154	100

BUN, serum creatinine, glucose, and electrolytes should be checked frequently. If neurological signs or symptoms supervene, then cerebral edema needs to be considered and appropriate adjustments made. The use of CT or MRI of the brain may be useful in the diagnosis of cerebral edema as a complication of correction therapy. An appreciation of maintenance fluid requirements and ongoing losses is necessary [2,16,17,25].

Chronic asymptomatic hypernatremia should be corrected slowly, 8–10 mEq/L over 24 hours or 0.5 mEq/L/h as a maximal rate over 48 hours, or even 72 hours. The use of oral and enteral fluids is preferred if possible [16]. Pitfalls in therapy include overly rapid correction of hypernatremia, hyperglycemia due to 5% dextrose in water (D5W) at rates >500 mL/h, failure to replace ongoing fluid and electrolyte losses, and inadequate clinical and laboratory follow-up [16]. It is reasonable to obtain neurological vital signs, intake, and output hourly. Monitoring of serum electrolytes, BUN, creatinine, and glucose every 2 hours initially for 24 hours then every 4–6 hours, or until appropriate correction of hypernatremia, should be carried out.

Formulae for hypernatremia management and infusate characteristics have been provided by Adrogué and Madias (see **Tables 9** and **12**) [1]. These formulae are most useful in the presence of pure water deficit and link therapy with water deficit. They provide the estimated effect of 1 L of infusate on serum sodium and are clinically useful. An example of the calculated water deficit and the use of these formulas can be found in **Appendices I** and **II**. An algorithm for the management of hypernatremia is provided in **Figure 4** [2,25].

Hypovolemic hypernatremia

The treatment of hypovolemic hypernatremia involves administration of hypotonic fluid. Isotonic saline may be necessary if circulatory compromise or signs of hypoperfusion – such as hypotension, orthostasis, or prerenal azotemia – exist. The water deficit should be calculated. The initial administration of 0.45% saline and 5% dextrose, in addition to oral water intake and replacement of the deficit and ongoing losses, should be carried out.

Hypervolemic hypernatremia

Since a patient with hypervolemic hypernatremia has hyperosmolality and an increase in total body sodium, the use of water replacement and diuretic therapy is necessary. Removal of sodium and addition of water is required. Loop diuretics, like furosemide, produce hypotonic urine with an approximate urine sodium concentration of 75 mEq/L, equivalent to half

Table 13. Treatment of central diabetes insipidus.
Reprinted from *Comprehensive Clinical Nephrology*, Johnson JR, Feehally J, editors. Chapter 9: Disorders of water metabolism, Berl T, Kumar S:9.1–9.20. Copyright 2004, with permission from Elsevier.

Disease	Drug	Dose	Dosage interval (hours)
Complete central diabetes insipidus	Desmopressin	10–20 μg intranasally 0.05 mg orally twice daily initially Titrate	12–24 12–24
Partial central diabetes insipidus	Desmopressin	10–20 μg intranasally 0.05 mg orally twice daily initially Titrate	12–24 12–24
	Vasopressin tannate	2–5 U intramuscularly	24–48
	Aqueous vasopressin	5–10 U subcutaneously	4–6
	Chlorpropamide	250–500 mg orally	24
	Clofibrate	500 mg orally	6 or 8
	Carbamazepine	400–600 mg orally	24

normal saline (NS). Therefore, diuretics alone may worsen hypernatremia if not given in conjunction with oral water, D5W, or D5 0.2% in water NS. The key factor is to ensure that intravenous fluids are hypotonic compared with the urine. Remember, the patient will also have insensible water loss and this must be accounted for [2,16,17,25]. Antagonism of aldosterone effects with spironolactone may be useful in patients with hyperaldosteronism or Cushing's syndrome. In severe acute cases in the presence of renal failure, cardiopulmonary disease, or hepatorenal disease with volume overload, acute hemodialysis with a low sodium dialysate (sodium 110 mEq/L) may be necessary [30,31].

Euvolemic hypernatremia

After the calculation of the water deficit, treatment with hypotonic fluid should begin. The formulae for management of hypernatremia are most useful here as there is a pure deficit of water. There are no controlled studies identifying the optimal fluid administration in hypernatremia; however, initial administration of D5 1/2 NS intravenously and oral water replacement is a good way to start. In the presence of circulatory compromise, initial treatment with 0.9% saline may be necessary [2]. Potassium losses and maintenance need to be repleted. In the presence of central diabetes insipidus, aqueous vasopressin (Pitressin; Monarch Pharmaceuticals, Bristol, TN, USA), at a dose of 5 units subcutaneously every 6 hours, should be used with careful follow-up of serum sodium to avoid hyponatremia [2,16,17].

Chronic therapy of complete or partial central diabetes insipidus consists of aqueous vasopressin, vasopressin tannate, and desmopressin, intranasally or orally (see **Table 13**). Therapy of partial diabetes insipidus includes chlorpropamide, clofibrate, and carbamazepine, which can enhance the effect of circulating ADH (see **Table 13**) [2,17]. The treatment of nephrogenic diabetes insipidus includes a low protein and sodium diet, thiazide diuretics, amiloride, and nonsteroidal anti-inflammatory drugs [17,27,28,32].

Vasopressin in the ICU

Vasopressin has recently been used for hemodynamic support of septic shock and vasodilatory shock caused by systemic inflammatory response syndrome [33]. Vasopressin has vasopressor, antidiuretic, hemostatic, and thermoregulatory effects. V_1 receptors, located in vascular smooth muscle, mediate vasoconstriction, and V_2 receptors mediate the effect of vasopressin on the renal CCD. In septic shock, vasopressin levels are low relative to other causes of hypotension. Acutely ill septic patients may have vasopressin insufficiency, as suggested by the loss of the pituitary bright spot in T1-weighted MRI images in one study [34]. Subpharmacologic vasopressin infusion at levels of 0.01–0.04 U/min can increase plasma vasopressin levels and decrease the dose requirement for other vasopressors. Urine output may increase. Pharmacologic doses of >0.04 U/min, giving plasma levels of >100 pg/mL, are associated with the negative effects of vasoconstriction on the renal, coronary, pulmonary, and mesenteric vasculature [33].

References

1. Adrogue HJ, Madias NE. Hyponatremia. *N Engl J Med* 2000;342:1581–9.
2. Berl T, Kumar S. Disorders of water metabolism. In: Johnson RJ, Freehally J, editors. *Comprehensive Clinical Nephrology*. London: Mosby 2000:9.1–9.20.
3. Berl T, Robertson GL. Pathophysiology of water metabolism. In: Brenner BM, editor. *The Kidney*. Philadelphia, PA: WB Saunders & Company, 2000:866–924.
4. Sterns RH, Ocdol H, Schrier RW et al. Hyponatremia: pathophysiology, diagnosis, and therapy. In: Narins RG, editor. *Clinical Disorders of Fluid and Electrolyte Metabolism*. New York, NY: McGraw-Hill, 1994:583–615.
5. Verbalis JG. Hyponatremia and hypoosmolar disorders. In: Greenberg A, editor. *Primer on Kidney Diseases*. San Diego, CA: Academic Press, 2001:57–63.
6. Musch W, Thimpont J, Vandervelde D et al. Combined fractional excretion of sodium and urea better predicts response to saline in hyponatremia than do usual clinical and biochemical parameters. *Am J Med* 1995;99:348–55.
7. Anderson RJ, Chung HM, Kluge R et al. Hyponatremia: a prospective analysis of its epidemiology and the pathogenetic role of vasopressin. *Ann Intern Med* 1985;102:164–8.
8. Soupart A, Decaux G. Therapeutic recommendations for management of severe hyponatremia: current concepts on pathogenesis and prevention of neurologic complications. *Clin Nephrol* 1996;46:149–69.
9. Gross P, Reimann D, Henschkowski J et al. Treatment of severe hyponatremia: conventional and novel aspects. *J Am Soc Nephrol* 2001;12(Suppl. 17):S10–14.
10. Oster JR, Singer I. Hyponatremia, hyposmolality, and hypotonicity: tables and fables. *Arch Intern Med* 1999;159:333–6.
11. Hillier TA, Abbott RD, Barrett EJ. Hyponatremia: evaluating the correction factor for hyperglycemia. *Am J Med* 1999;106:399–403.
12. Katz MA. Hyperglycemia-induced hyponatremia – calculation of expected serum sodium depression. *N Engl J Med* 1973;289:843–4.
13. Shichiri M, Shinoda T, Kijima Y et al. Renal handling of urate in the syndrome of inappropriate secretion of antidiuretic hormone. *Arch Intern Med* 1985;145:2045–7.
14. Coursin DB, Wood KE. Corticosteroid supplementation for adrenal insufficiency. *JAMA* 2002;287:236–40.
15. Oya S, Tsutsumi K, Ueki K et al. Reinduction of hyponatremia to treat central pontine myelinolysis. *Neurology* 2001;57:1931–2.
16. Adrogue HJ, Madias NE. Hypernatremia. *N Engl J Med* 2000;342:1493–9.
17. Palevsky PM. Hypernatremia. In: Greenberg A, Ed. *Primer on Kidney Diseases*. San Diego, CA: Academic Press, 2001:64–71.
18. Snyder NA, Feigal DW, Arieff AI. Hypernatremia in elderly patients. A heterogeneous, morbid, and iatrogenic entity. *Ann Intern Med* 1987;107:309–19.
19. Goldszer RC, Coodley EL. Survival with severe hypernatremia. *Arch Intern Med* 1979;139:936–7.
20. Polderman KH, Schreuder WO, Strack van Schijndel RJ et al. Hypernatremia in the intensive care unit: an indicator of quality of care? *Crit Care Med* 1999;27:1105–8.

21. Kahn T. Hypernatremia with edema. *Arch Intern Med* 1999;159:93–8.

22. Palevsky PM, Bhagrath R, Greenberg A. Hypernatremia in hospitalized patients. *Ann Intern Med* 1996;124:197–203.

23. Moder KG, Hurley DL. Fatal hypernatremia from exogenous salt intake: report of a case and review of the literature. *Mayo Clin Proc* 1990;65:1587–94.

24. Lee JH, Arcinue E, Ross BD. Brief report: organic osmolytes in the brain of an infant with hypernatremia. *N Engl J Med* 1994;331:439–42.

25. Berl T, Robertson G. Pathophysiology of water metabolism. In: Brenner BM, editor. *The Kidney*. Philadelphia, PA: WB Saunders & Company, 2000:866–924.

26. Felig P, Johnson C, Levitt M et al. Hypernatremia induced by maximal exercise. *JAMA* 1982;248:1209–11.

27. Bichet DG. Nephrogenic diabetes insipidus. *Am J Med* 1998;105:431–42.

28. Bichet DG, Oksche A, Rosenthal W. Congenital nephrogenic diabetes insipidus. *J Am Soc Nephrol* 1997;8:1951–8.

29. Durr JA, Hoggard JG, Hunt JM et al. Diabetes insipidus in pregnancy associated with abnormally high circulating vasopressinase activity. *N Engl J Med* 1987;316:1070–4.

30. Pazmino PA, Pazmino BP. Treatment of acute hypernatremia with hemodialysis. *Am J Nephrol* 1993;13:260–5.

31. Yang CW, Kim YS, Park IS et al. Treatment of severe acute hypernatremia and renal failure by hemodialysis. *Nephron* 1995;70:372–3.

32. Alon U, Chan JC. Hydrochlorothiazide-amiloride in the treatment of congenital nephrogenic diabetes insipidus. *Am J Nephrol* 1985;5:9–13.

33. Holmes CL, Patel BM, Russell JA et al. Physiology of vasopressin relevant to management of septic shock. *Chest* 2001;120:989–1002.

34. Sharshar T, Carlier R, Blanchard A et al. Depletion of neurohypophyseal content of vasopressin in septic shock. *Crit Care Med* 2002;30:497–500.

Part 3: Edema

Richard N Hellman

Definition

Edema is defined as an accumulation of excess fluid in the interstitial spaces. Edema is due to an imbalance of membrane permeability and hydrostatic and oncotic forces, and it can be either generalized or localized. Generalized edema can be physiologically classified as edema due to reduced oncotic pressure, impaired lymphatic drainage, increased capillary permeability, increased hydrostatic pressure, or increased blood volume. Increased blood volume can occur with decreased or increased effective arterial volume. Edema impairs tissue oxygenation and may promote further edema formation. Edema is most often a manifestation of increased extracellular fluid (ECF) volume [1].

Causes of edema in the ICU patient

The major causes of edema in the intensive care unit are heart failure, renal failure, and liver failure, or a combination of these in the case of multiple organ dysfunction syndrome (MODS). Additional causes of edema are decreased muscle pump activity, mechanical ventilation, organ edema, acute peripheral vasodilatation, cardiodepression, protein extravasation, and renal vascular constriction and/or obstruction. Unusual causes of edema include hypothyroidism with myxedema and prescription of medications such as dihydropyridine calcium-channel blockers for hypertension [2].

Diuretic therapy

Edema is a manifestation of increased ECF volume and is associated with pathologic renal sodium retention or impaired excretion in patients with congestive heart failure (CHF), renal failure, cirrhosis, and nephrotic syndrome. Diuretics, which increase renal sodium and water excretion, are therefore important in the management of the volume-overloaded patient when sodium restriction alone is unsuccessful [1].

The purpose of **Part 3** is to describe the use of diuretic therapy in acute and chronic kidney disease (CKD), nephrotic syndrome, cirrhosis, and CHF. The use of diuretics for non-edematous conditions will not be discussed.

General measures in the management of edema are sodium restriction (dietary, intravenous [IV] fluid, and total parenteral nutrition [TPN]), appropriate water restriction for hyponatremia, appropriate water repletion for hypernatremia, oxygen therapy if the patient is hypoxemic, and an initial trial of bed rest (see **Section 2, Part 2.**) The goals of diuretic therapy should be identified before treatment onset and careful follow-up of weight, urine output, total intake and output, blood urea nitrogen (BUN), serum creatinine, electrolytes, calcium, phosphorus, albumin, and magnesium should be performed on all patients receiving diuretic therapy [1].

All diuretics except spironolactone reach the renal tubular luminal transport sites through the tubular fluid; all but osmotic diuretics are actively secreted into the urine by proximal renal tubular cells. Glomerular filtration can be limited by binding of the diuretic to proteins. Further reduction in the efficacy of diuretic can be caused by tolerance to the drug. Diuretic tolerance occurs in two forms: that related to volume depletion, and that which occurs due to increased segmental tubular sodium reabsorption. The latter form of resistance can be counteracted using a loop diuretic acting on the thick ascending limb (TAL) and a thiazide diuretic acting on the cortical diluting segment to establish total distal blockade. Nonsteroidal anti-inflammatory drugs, excessive sodium intake, and noncompliance with a diuretic regimen can all impair the usefulness of diuretics [3,4].

Diuretics in renal failure

Loop diuretics are the most powerful available and are the diuretics of choice in renal failure. The maximal renal response to a loop diuretic is excretion of 20% of the filtered load of sodium. Decreased glomerular filtration rate (GFR) leads to decreased delivery of loop diuretic to the TAL, thus reducing the diuretic response and creating the need for higher doses of therapy. Therapeutic regimens for the use of loop diuretics in renal insufficiency, nephrotic syndrome, cirrhosis, and CHF are listed in **Table 1** [3,4].

Acute renal failure

Restoration of perfusion pressure and hemodynamics, normalization of volume status, and exclusion of post- and prerenal azotemia are the first steps in the approach to the patient with oliguric acute renal failure (ARF). High-dose loop diuretics are used in an attempt to convert an oliguric into a non-oliguric ARF, but there is no compelling evidence to show that loop diuretics can forestall the development of ARF or prevent ARF in high-risk situations such as IV contrast administration in patients with impaired renal function. Furosemide is associated with a worse outcome in the prevention of IV contrast nephropathy in patients with underlying renal impairment when compared with volume expansion alone [5]. A recent observational study suggested increased all-cause mortality and nonrecovery of renal function in critically ill patients with ARF who were treated with diuretic therapy [6].

The usual clinical approach to diuretic therapy in ARF is a trial of IV furosemide either as a single dose or as an infusion with a follow-up analysis of urine output. An initial dose of furosemide is given and, if there is no response in 2–4 hours, then a further 100–200 mg IV dose of furosemide is given. If there is still no diuretic effect, addition of a thiazide such as metolazone at 5–10 mg orally or chlorothiazide 500 mg IV to the diuretic regimen can facilitate total distal tubule blockade. Some nephrologists use up to 500 mg of furosemide or 200 mg of torsemide, although the maximal IV bolus response to furosemide occurs with 200 mg of the drug. Loop diuretics (torsemide or bumetanide) may be used in place of furosemide. Continuous IV infusion of a loop diuretic (see **Table 2**) after an initial loading dose may confer a better diuretic response than a bolus dose of a loop diuretic [3,4,7,8].

Table 1. Therapeutic regimens for loop diuretics in patients with diminished responses to initial therapy.

[a]Preserved renal function is defined as a creatinine clearance of more than 75 mL/min; [b]If the maximal dose is reached without an adequate response, a thiazide diuretic should be administered as adjunctive therapy with the dose determined according to renal function, and alternative treatment of the primary disease should be considered.

Factor	Renal insufficiency		Preserved renal function[a]		
	Moderate	**Severe**	**Nephrotic syndrome**	**Cirrhosis**	**Congestive heart failure**
Mechanism of diminished response	Impaired delivery to site of action		Diminished nephron response, binding of diuretic to urinary protein	Diminished nephron response	Diminished nephron response
Therapeutic approach	Administration of sufficiently high dose to attain diuretic at site of action		Administration of sufficiently high dose to attain effective amount of unbound diuretic at site of action, more frequent administration of effective dose	More frequent administration of effective dose	More frequent administration of effective dose
Maximal intravenous dose (mg)[b]					
Furosemide	80–160	160–200	80–120	40	40–80
Bumetanide	4–8	8–10	2–3	1	1–2
Torsemide	20–50	50–100	20–50	10	10–20

Table 2. Doses for continuous intravenous infusion of loop diuretics.

[a]Before the infusion rate is increased, the loading dose should be administered again.

Diuretic	Intravenous loading dose (mg)	Infusion rate[a] (mg/h)		
		Creatinine clearance <25 mL/min	**Creatinine clearance 25–75 mL/min**	**Creatinine clearance >75 mL/min**
Furosemide	40	20 then 40	10 then 20	10
Bumetanide	1	1 then 2	0.5 then 1	0.5
Torsemide	20	10 then 20	5 then 10	5

The use of albumin infusion with a loop diuretic probably does not increase clinical diuresis in most patients but may be considered in those with profound hypoalbuminemia (serum albumin <2 g/dL) [9,10]. BUN, serum creatinine, electrolytes, calcium, phosphorus, and magnesium tests should be performed on all patients at least daily to preempt diuretic complications (see **Table 3**) [1–4,11,12]. If diuresis cannot be established and the patient remains oliguric with rising serum creatinine, diuretics should be discontinued, and hemodialysis or continuous renal replacement therapy (CRRT) will be necessary

Table 3. Complications of diuretic therapy.

[a]Eg, spironolactone, acetazolamide.

Fluid, electrolyte, and acid–base abnormalities	Metabolic complications	Other side effects
Extracellular volume depletion	Hyperuricemia	Ototoxicity
Hyponatremia	Hyperglycemia	Impotence
Hypokalemia	Hyperlipidemia	Gynecomastia
Hypomagnesemia		Osteomalacia
Hypercalcemia		Hypersensitivity reactions
Metabolic alkalosis		Renal cell cancer
Metabolic acidosis[a]		Pancreatitis

(see **Sections 3** and **4**). Osmotic diuretics such as mannitol usually do not have a place in the management of ARF except in the prevention of myoglobinuric ARF. Similarly, carbonic anhydrase inhibitors such as acetazolamide and potassium-sparing diuretics are generally not used in ARF due to weak diuretic effect, metabolic acidosis, and the potential for hyperkalemia.

Complications of diuretic therapy

The complications of diuretic therapy are listed in **Table 3**. Ototoxicity has been seen with high-dose furosemide infusion; therefore, furosemide doses should be limited to an infusion of 200 mg over 1–2 hours, or infusion at rates of <4 mg/min [1–4,11,12].

Chronic kidney disease

The bioavailability of loop diuretics does not differ between normal subjects and patients with renal insufficiency. The IV doses of bumetanide and torsemide are equivalent to the oral doses, but the maximal oral dose of furosemide is twice that of the IV dose. Torsemide and bumetanide have better and more predictable bioavailability when compared to furosemide. Furosemide should be given at least twice a day in order to minimize the resistance effect.

The initial approach to the CKD patient is sodium restriction (only 3 g/day) and the initiation of a loop diuretic. A starting dose of furosemide or an equivalent is 40 mg twice daily, with doubling of the dose until appropriate diuretic response is reached (maximum dose is 160–200 mg three times a day). A thiazide diuretic such as metolazone at 5–10 mg/day can be added if there is inadequate diuresis. A 24-hour urine sodium test can be helpful in monitoring for diuretic resistance and should be at a level of <100 mEq/day. Excessive diuresis should be avoided, and the "push–pull" relationship between CHF and renal insufficiency is often a delicate balance in the ICU patient.

Diuretics in nephrotic syndrome

The treatment approach to nephrotic syndrome is similar to that for CKD (see **Table 1**). Sodium restriction and loop diuretics, with or without thiazide, are the usual treatments of choice. Definitive treatment of the underlying cause of nephrotic syndrome if available and the use of angiotensin-converting enzyme (ACE) inhibitors and/or angiotensin receptor blockers (ARBs) will reduce proteinuria [13]. In refractory NS with profound albuminemia (serum albumin <2 g/dL), a trial of high-dose furosemide (200 mg) and albumin (25 g) is recommended, although two studies have cast some doubt on this strategy [9,10]. In severe refractory nephrotic syndrome, CRRT may be necessary (see **Section 4**).

Diuretics in cirrhosis

General procedures in the treatment of cirrhotic edema are dietary sodium restriction (90 mEq [1–3 g] Na^+/day) and the restriction of oral fluid intake to <600–1,000 mL/day in the presence of hyponatremia. Regular follow-up of weight, intake and output, BUN, creatinine, electrolytes, and serum albumin is necessary.

Spironolactone is the diuretic of choice at a starting dose of 50 mg/day if urinary sodium is <30 mEq/L. Additional use of either furosemide or hydrochlorothiazide (25–50 mg/day) or metolazone (2.5–10 mg/day) is required if urinary sodium is >10–30 mEq/L. If furosemide is used, the ratio should be 40 mg of furosemide to 100 mg of spironolactone.

If urinary sodium is <10 mEq/L in the presence of edema and ascites, large-volume paracentesis with albumin infusion volume expansion (8 g/L of ascites fluid removed) is indicated. This has been shown to lower morbidity from hyponatremia, renal impairment, and hepatic encephalopathy.

Target diuresis is a weight loss of 0.5 kg/day in the presence of ascites alone, and 1 kg/day in patients with peripheral edema [2,3,14].

Refractory ascites is seen in 10%–20% of patients with cirrhosis. Treatment options are repeated large-volume paracentesis with albumin infusion, peritoneovenous shunt, and transjugular intrahepatic portosystemic shunt (TIPS) placement.

Hepatorenal syndrome (HRS) is defined as functional renal failure in patients with cirrhosis and ascites. It is characterized by a rising serum creatinine, relative hyperosmolality of the urine, and a urine sodium level <10 mEq/L. The treatment for HRS is orthotopic liver transplantation, but interim support with CRRT or liver dialysis may be necessary to prepare the patient for this procedure [2,3,14].

Diuretics in congestive heart failure

Improvement of cardiac pump function and hemodynamics are the goals of treatment in the case of edema associated with CHF. General treatment measures include sodium restriction, appropriate water restriction if hyponatremia is present, oxygenation (partial pressure of O_2>60 mm Hg), and the correction of anemia. Correction of anemia in patients with mild CKD and CHF can reduce diuretic requirements and the number of hospital admissions [15].

Laboratory assessment of BUN, creatinine, electrolytes, calcium, phosphorus, and albumin should be performed regularly, and serum potassium should be maintained at a normal level (4 mEq/L). Brain natriuretic peptide (BNP) levels may be measured as an initial diagnostic test and in follow-up investigations (BNP levels are raised in patients with CHF and increased intravascular volume), and can be useful in the management of CHF [16].

The standard of care for patients with CHF includes spironolactone (25 mg/day), ACE inhibitor, loop diuretic and/or β-blockers (such as metoprolol and carvedilol). Other therapeutic options include digoxin for symptom relief, and ARBs and hydralazine plus nitrates in patients who are intolerant to ACE inhibitors. Mild CHF, in the absence of renal failure, should be managed with hydrochlorothiazide, 25–50 mg/day. Loop diuretics may be necessary if there is inadequate diuretic response or renal insufficiency. Response to loop diuretics is generally more vigorous in CHF than nephrotic syndrome or renal failure. Consequently, lower doses of furosemide should be used due to concerns about over-diuresis, especially with combinations of loop diuretics and thiazides [1–3,16–19]. In the presence of renal insufficiency, potassium-sparing diuretics like spironolactone, ACE inhibitors, ARBs, and non-selective β-blockers may worsen renal function and cause hyperkalemia (see **Section 2, Part 4**).

In ICU patients with CHF and edema, the following treatments may be necessary: blood pressure control, arrhythmia management, inotropic agents and pressors (eg, dobutamine and dopamine), and α-atrial natriuretic peptide. Treatment of profound cardiomyopathy may include placement of an intra-aortic balloon pump or ventricular assist device, and CRRT support.

References

1. Ellison D. Edema and the clinical use of diuretics. In: Greenberg A, Coffman TM, editors. *Primer on Kidney Diseases*. 3rd ed. San Diego, CA: Academic Press, 2001:116–26.
2. Edema: pathophysiology and therapy. The Telesio Conference. Consenza, Italy, October 21–22, 1996. Proceedings. *Kidney Int Suppl* 1997;59:S1–134.
3. Brater DC. Diuretic therapy. *N Engl J Med* 1998;339:387–95.
4. Brater DC. Pharmacology of diuretics. *Am J Med Sci* 2000;319:38–50.
5. Solomon R, Werner C, Mann D et al. Effects of saline, mannitol, and furosemide to prevent acute decreases in renal function induced by radiocontrast agents. *N Engl J Med* 1994;331:1416–20.
6. Mehta RL, Pascual MT, Soroko S et al. Diuretics, mortality, and nonrecovery of renal function in acute renal failure. *JAMA* 2002;288:2547–53.
7. Fliser D, Schroter M, Neubeck M et al. Coadministration of thiazides increases the efficacy of loop diuretics even in patients with advanced renal failure. *Kidney Int* 1994;46:482–8.
8. Boesken WH, Kult J. High-dose torasemide, given once daily intravenously for one week, in patients with advanced chronic renal failure. *Clin Nephrol* 1997;48:22–8.
9. Chalasani N, Gorski JC, Horlander JC Sr et al. Effects of albumin/furosemide mixtures on responses to furosemide in hypoalbuminemic patients. *J Am Soc Nephrol* 2001;12:1010–6.
10. Agarwal R, Gorski JC, Sundblad K et al. Urinary protein binding does not affect response to furosemide in patients with nephrotic syndrome. *J Am Soc Nephrol* 2000;11:1100–5.
11. Greenberg A. Diuretic complications. *Am J Med Sci* 2000;319(1):10–24.
12. Gallagher KL, Jones JK. Furosemide-induced ototoxicity. *Ann Intern Med* 1979;91:744–5.
13. Remuzzi G, Ruggenenti P, Perico N. Chronic renal diseases: renoprotective benefits of renin-angiotensin system inhibition. *Ann Intern Med* 2002;136:604–15.
14. Menon KV, Kamath PS. Managing the complications of cirrhosis. *Mayo Clin Proc* 2000;75:501–9.
15. Silverberg DS, Wexler D, Sheps D et al. The effect of correction of mild anemia in severe, resistant congestive heart failure using subcutaneous erythropoietin and intravenous iron: a randomized controlled study. *J Am Coll Cardiol* 2001;37:1775–80.

16. Levin ER, Gardner DG, Samson WK. Natriuretic peptides. *N Engl J Med* 1998;339:321–8.

17. Kasper EK. What's new in the ACC/AHA guidelines for the evaluation and management of chronic heart failure in adults. *Adv Stud Med* 2003;3:14–21.

18. Hunt SA, Baker DW, Chin MH et al. ACC/AHA guidelines for the evaluation and management of chronic heart failure in the adult: executive summary. A report of the American College of Cardiology/American Heart Association Task Force on Practice Guidelines (Committee to revise the 1995 Guidelines for the Evaluation and Management of Heart Failure). *J Am Coll Cardiol* 2001;38:2101–13.

19. Weber KT. Aldosterone in congestive heart failure. *N Engl J Med* 2001;345:1689–97.

Part 4: Disorders of potassium metabolism

Richard N Hellman

Introduction

Potassium (K^+) is the major intracellular cation and the second most abundant cation in the body. Ninety-eight percent of K^+ in the body is intracellular. Two systems regulate K^+ homeostasis: the first regulates shifts between intracellular and extracellular K^+ to maintain a constant extracellular K^+ concentration, and the second regulates K^+ excretion, mainly by the kidneys and, to a lesser extent, the intestine and sweat glands [1]. The transcellular K^+ concentration gradient is maintained by the activity of the cellular sodium (Na^+)–K^+-ATPase and is responsible for resting cell membrane potential, neuromuscular excitability, and cardiac pacemaker function [1,2].

Serum K^+ is maintained at a constant level of ≈4 mmol/L (≈4 mEq/L) and a normal range of 3.5–5.5 mmol/L. Serum K^+ is 0.5–0.9 mmol/L higher than plasma K^+.

Potassium balance

Factors responsible for maintenance of the extracellular fluid (ECF) K^+ concentration can be categorized into physiological factors and pathological factors (**Figure 1**) [1,3,4]. Physiological factors including Na^+–K^+-ATPase activity, insulin, β_2-adrenergic agonist activity catecholamines, aldosterone, thyroid hormone, and plasma K^+ concentration all promote cellular K^+ entry, lowering serum K^+; conversely, α-receptor stimulation (eg, epinephrine) and exercise increase serum K^+. Insulin, independent of its effect on blood glucose, increases Na^+–K^+-ATPase activity, thereby promoting skeletal muscle and hepatic uptake of K^+ and reducing the serum K^+ concentration [5].

Pathologic factors that increase plasma K^+ include cell lysis, plasma hyperosmolality, and acidosis. Cells respond to a decrease in serum pH with an increase in cellular uptake of protons (H^+): this leads to an efflux of K^+ into the ECF to preserve electrical neutrality. Generally, for each 0.1 unit decrease in pH there is a 0.6 mEq/L increase in serum K^+. Organic acidosis, such as lactic acidosis, is associated with less hyperkalemia as transmembrane diffusion of both H^+ and negatively charged lactate preserves electrical neutrality [6]. Alkalosis, on the other hand, causes hypokalemia: efflux of H^+ from the intracellular fluid (ICF) into the ECF is associated with a counterbalancing influx of K^+.

Aldosterone can increase cellular uptake of K^+, and may have a role independent of its actions on the kidney. The primary action of aldosterone is on the kidney, where it increases Na^+–K^+-ATPase activity and increases the number of apical epithelial Na^+ and K^+ channels in the principal cells of the cortical collecting duct, thereby leading to increased urinary K^+. The major factors regulating aldosterone secretion are angiotensin II and K^+. Hyperkalemia stimulates

Figure 1. Potassium balance. Ninety-eight percent of potassium (K^+) is in the intracellular fluid (ICF) and 2% is in the extracellular fluid (ECF). Physiologic and pathologic factors influencing K^+ shifts between ECF and ICF are listed.

Reproduced with permission from Sterns RH, Cox M, Feig PU et al. Internal potassium balance and the control of the plasma potassium concentration. *Medicine* 1981;60:339–54.

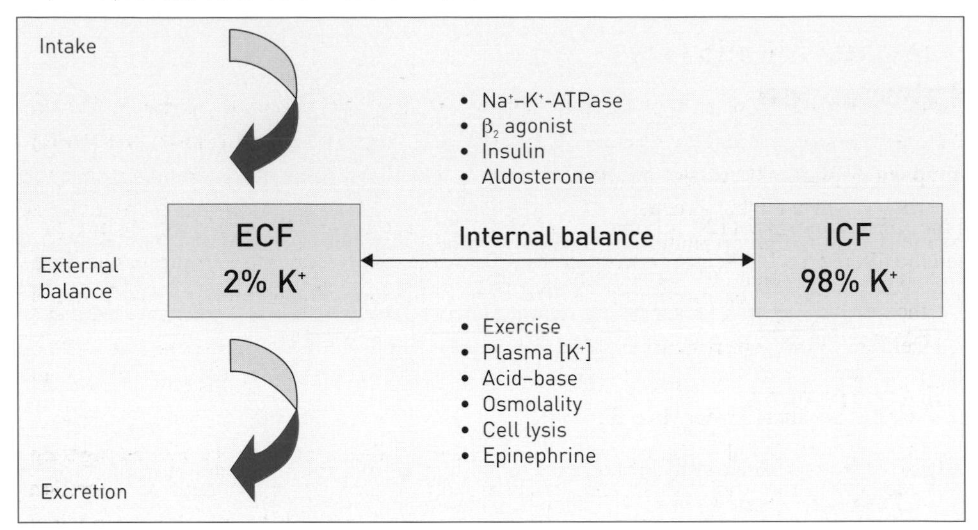

aldosterone production, leading to increased renal K^+ excretion [1,6,7]. Corticotropin can modulate aldosterone secretion but this is not important under normal physiologic conditions. However, in congestive heart failure the levels of corticotropin may be chronically increased and may have an impact on aldosterone production and secretion [2,3,7,8].

Relationship between serum K^+ and total body K^+

Since only 2% of K^+ is extracellular, measurements of serum or plasma K^+ can only provide an imprecise indicator of total body K^+ stores. Indeed, large deficits of total body K^+ may be present despite only small declines in serum K^+. It is important to distinguish between hypokalemia and K^+ deficiency where there is a deficit of total body K^+ due to negative K^+ balance. It is possible to be K^+ deficient with normokalemia, and even with hyperkalemia. In patients with diabetic ketoacidosis (DKA), hyperosmolality, due to hyperglycemia, acidosis, and insulin deficiency can lead to normokalemia or hyperkalemia despite the patient having a negative K^+ balance as a result of osmotic diuresis. Treatment with insulin and fluids corrects the acidosis, hyperglycemia, and hyperosmolality, and unmasks the underlying K^+ deficit. DKA patients often require K^+ replacement during correction of their underlying disturbances.

Renal handling of potassium

Although the kidney has the ability to conserve K^+ in the face of reduced intake, and increase excretion in the presence of a K^+ load, renal adaptation to K^+ deficiency is not as complete or prompt as that due to sodium deficiency. In the presence of K^+ depletion, only 1% of the filtered load of K^+ is excreted, and urinary K^+ levels can fall to 5–10 mEq/L; in the presence of a high or normal K^+ diet, between 15%–80% of the filtered load is excreted, and urinary K^+

levels can increase to 100 mEq/L [1,2,7,8]. This renal adaptation is gradual, taking hours to days, whereas cellular shifts are instantaneous.

Potassium transport by the nephron

Glomerular filtration rate

A total of 10%–20% of serum K^+ is protein bound, and the remainder is freely filtered at the glomerulus. The filtered load of K^+ is equal to the glomerular filtration rate (GFR) multiplied by plasma K^+ concentration.

If the GFR is normal (120 mL/min or 172.8 L/day), and serum K^+ levels are 4.0 mEq/L, then the filtered load of K^+ is 692 mEq/day or 590 mEq/day when corrected for protein binding. The average fractional excretion of K^+ is 10%–20% of the filtered load, yielding 70–120 mmol K^+ excretion daily [3].

Tubular function

A total of 10%–15% of the filtered load of K^+ reaches the distal tubule. Since 90% of ingested K^+ is excreted in the urine, K^+ secretion clearly plays a major role in K^+ balance. Secretion and reabsorption of K^+ occur in the cortical collecting tubule. Both principal cells and intercalated cells can reabsorb K^+ but only principal cells can secrete K^+ [7]. Aldosterone, plasma K^+, tubular fluid sodium, tubular fluid flow rate, non-reabsorbable anion, and acid-base status are the major factors determining K^+ secretion by the principal cells of the cortical collecting duct. In addition, anything that increases luminal negativity – such as a nonreabsorbable anion – will favor K^+ secretion. Diuretics can increase distal nephron Na^+ delivery and increase urinary flow rate – factors that favor K^+ secretion. Conversely, blocking the apical Na^+ channel (eg, with drugs such as amiloride, trimethoprim, or pentamidine) will decrease K^+ secretion and favor the development of hyperkalemia, especially in the presence of underlying renal dysfunction [3,7,9].

Adaptation in renal failure

In the presence of chronic kidney disease (CKD), the fractional excretion of K^+ per nephron unit is increased due to increased Na^+–K^+-ATPase activity in cortical collecting-duct cells. Serum aldosterone levels are often elevated in patients with CKD, and elevated serum aldosterone and serum K^+ stimulate K^+ excretion. Overt hyperkalemia is not usually seen until creatinine clearances are <10–15 mL/min [10]. However, there is a subgroup of patients with either diabetic nephropathy or interstitial nephritis that can have significant hyperkalemia and hyperchloremic metabolic acidosis (type IV renal tubular acidosis) due to hyporenin–hypoaldosterone syndromes. The use of drugs that reduce aldosterone (eg, nonsteroidal anti-inflammatory drugs [NSAIDs] and angiotensin-converting enzyme [ACE] inhibitors), block aldosterone's effects (eg, spironolactone), block the apical Na^+ channel (eg, trimethoprim), or block cellular K^+ uptake (eg, non-selective β-blockers such as propranolol) can lead to hyperkalemia in patients with CKD. Treatment of diabetic patients with congestive heart failure and mild CKD (serum creatinine >1.5–2.0 mg/dL) frequently

Table 1. Useful laboratory tests for K^+ disorders.
ECG: electrocardiogram.

Serum electrolytes
Serum creatinine
Serum pH
Serum Mg^{2+}
Spot serum aldosterone:renin ratio
ECG
Spot urine K^+>20 or <20 mEq/L
24-hour urinary K^+
Fractional excretion of K^+

involves a cocktail of aldosterone antagonist, β-blocker, and ACE inhibitor. This regimen may be associated with significant hyperkalemia, and its use requires frequent monitoring of electrolytes and renal function [1–3,9,11].

Evaluation of the patient with a potassium disorder

Serum K^+ must be looked at in the context of overall renal function, as measured by the calculated creatinine clearance, acid–base status, and volume status of the patient (see **Table 1**). It is important to distinguish between hypokalemia and hyperkalemia, and between a net total body deficit and excess of K^+. Pseudohyperkalemia, as occurs in profound leukocytosis, thrombocytosis, or spurious hyperkalemia, must be ruled out [1,7].

A careful history and physical examination must be conducted, with due attention given to underlying disease states, medications, and "remedies" used by the patient. The use of salt substitute (potassium chloride [KCl]) may be a cause of hyperkalemia in patients with CKD. NSAIDs can block prostaglandin release and reduce renin, and subsequently aldosterone levels, and thereby cause hyperkalemia in patients.

Measurement of the fractional excretion of K^+ (FEK) is useful in evaluating K^+ disorders, particularly hypokalemia. It is calculated as follows from a random urine sample:

$$\frac{[U_K/P_K]}{[U_{CR}/P_{CR}]} \times 100 = \text{FEK}$$

(Where U_K is urine potassium, P_K is plasma or serum potassium, U_{CR} is urine creatinine, and P_{CR} is plasma creatinine.) A person with normal renal function on an average potassium diet (70–100 mEq/day) has an FEK of 10%.

In the presence of a K^+ deficit, urinary K^+ levels and the FEK should be low; in the presence of K^+ loading, they should be elevated. If a patient has a low serum K^+ and a low urinary K^+ or low FEK then an extrarenal source of K^+ loss should be sought. In a patient with hypokalemia, a urinary K^+ of <20 mEq/day is suggestive of an extrarenal etiology of the hypokalemia, whilst a urinary K^+ of >20 mEq/day suggests a renal etiology. Ideally, testing needs to be completed before attempts are made to correct the hypokalemia or hyperkalemia, and should not be confounded by diuretic use [8].

Table 2. Causes of hypokalemia.

HTN: hypertension; RTA: renal tubular acidosis.

Extrarenal K^+ losses	Vomiting Diarrhea
Urinary K^+ losses	Diuretics Osmotic diuresis
Hypokalemia with hypertension	Primary aldosteronism Glucocorticoid-responsive HTN Malignant HTN Renovascular HTN Renin-secreting tumor HTN with diuretic R_x Liddle's syndrome 11β-hydroxysteroid dehydrogenase deficiency (genetic) Drug induced Chewing tobacco, licorice, some French wines Congenital adrenal hyperplasia
Hypokalemia with normal blood pressure	Distal RTA (type I) Proximal RTA (type II) Bartter's syndrome Gitelman's syndrome Hypomagnesemia (cisplatinum, alcoholism, diuretics)
Hypokalemia due to potassium shifts	Insulin administration Catecholamine excess Familial periodic paralysis Thyrotoxic hypokalemic paralysis
Inadequate intake	Low K^+ diet

Spot serum aldosterone:renin ratio

The presence of hypokalemia and hypertension, in addition to an increased FEK, can indicate a mineralocorticoid excess syndrome such as primary hyperaldosteronism. A spot serum sample for aldosterone and renin is a useful screening tool in this situation. This is based on the premise that autonomous production of aldosterone – by either an adenoma or hyperplasia – will suppress renin production due to volume expansion. Therefore, the serum aldosterone:renin ratio will be high in primary aldosteronism (>30–50). In secondary hyperaldosteronism (eg, following volume depletion), levels of both renin and aldosterone will be increased and the aldosterone:renin ratio will not be elevated [7,8].

Hypokalemia

Definition

Hypokalemia is defined as a serum K^+ level of <3.5 mEq/L (<3.5 mmol/L). It is important to distinguish between hypokalemia and a true deficit in TBK.

Table 3. Drug-induced hypokalemia.

Hypokalemia due to transcellular potassium shift	Hypokalemia due to increased renal potassium loss	Hypokalemia due to excess potassium loss in stool
β_2-adrenergic agonists - Epinephrine Decongestants - Pseudoephedrine - Phenylpropanolamine Bronchodilators - Albuterol - Terbutaline - Pirbuterol - Isoetharine - Fenoterol - Ephedrine - Isoproterenol - Metaproterenol Tocolytic agents - Ritodrine - Nylidrin Theophylline Caffeine Verapamil intoxication Chloroquine intoxication Insulin overdose	Diuretics - Acetazolamide - Thiazides - Chlorthalidone - Indapamide - Metolazone - Quinethazone - Bumetanide - Ethacrynic acid - Furosemide - Torsemide Mineralocorticoids - Fludrocortisone Substances with mineralocorticoid effects - Licorice - Carbenoxolone - Gossypol High-dose glucocorticoids High-dose antibiotics - Penicillin - Nafcillin - Ampicillin - Carbenicillin Drugs associated with magnesium depletion - Aminoglycosides - Cisplatin - Foscarnet Amphotericin B	Phenolphthalein Sodium polystyrene sulfonate

Demography

Hypokalemia is a common finding in clinical practice, being seen in 20% of hospitalized patients and in 10%–40% of patients on thiazide diuretics. In post-myocardial infarction patients or those with coronary artery disease, maintaining serum K^+ in the range of 3.6–5.1 mEq/L may reduce the risk of ventricular arrhythmias [6–8,12]. A goal serum K^+ level of ≥4 mEq/L is indicated in patients with cardiac arrhythmias.

Etiologies

The major categories in the differential diagnosis of hypokalemia are poor K^+ intake – which is rare – extrarenal losses due to nausea and vomiting, renal losses, and shifts in K^+ from ECF to ICF. Insulin administration, catecholamines, acid–base status, and hypokalemic periodic paralysis (a sporadic or autosomal-dominant abnormality of muscle tissue) can cause hypokalemia-related ECF to ICF shifts (see **Table 2**) [7].

Diuretics cause hypokalemia by increasing cortical collecting duct (CCD) tubular flow rates and tubular Na^+ levels, and are often associated with metabolic alkalosis and secondary

Table 4. Physiological consequences of hypokalemia.

ECG: electrocardiogram; U_{MAX}: maximum urine concentrating ability.
Reproduced with permission from Gabow PA, Peterson LN. Disorders of potassium metabolism. In: *Renal and Electrolyte Disorders*, Second Edition. Schrier RW, editor.

Neuromuscular	Rhabdomyolysis Muscle cramps Ileus Weakness: quadriparesis or quadriplegia Autonomic insufficiency: orthostatic hypotension Tetany
Renal	Polyuria and polydipsia Decreased U_{MAX} Increased renal ammonia production Edema and sodium retention Hypokalemic nephropathy and cysts
Hormonal	Decreased aldosterone secretion Decreased insulin release Altered prostaglandin synthesis
Metabolic	Abnormal carbohydrate metabolism Negative nitrogen balance Encephalopathy in patients with liver disease
Cardiac	Vasoconstriction and hypertension Myocardial cell necrosis U waves on ECG Digitalis toxicity

hyperaldosteronism. Hypokalemia with hypertension may be due to mineralocorticoid excess syndrome (either primary or secondary) or associated with a specific tubular defect such as Liddle's syndrome. Liddle's syndrome is a rare autosomal-dominant disorder associated with increased CCD apical Na^+ channel sodium absorption and, therefore, K^+ secretion. Hypokalemia associated with normotension is seen with renal tubular acidosis (RTA types I and II), hypomagnesemia, and Bartter's and Gitelman's syndromes. Bartter's syndrome is an inherited tubular disorder where there is a defect in the Na^+–K^+–$2Cl^-$ transporter in the thick ascending limb of the loop of Henle. These patients behave as if they are on loop diuretic such as furosemide. Gitelman's syndrome patients act as if they are on chronic thiazide diuretic therapy [13]. Surreptitious use of either loop diuretic or thiazide diuretic can be mistaken for these syndromes [14]. Drugs can also cause hypokalemia via enhanced transcellular shifts, renal losses, and extrarenal losses (**Table 3**).

Physiological consequences

The physiological consequences of hypokalemia (**Table 4**), particularly those due to cardiac arrhythmias and neuromuscular weakness, signal a need for prompt treatment.

Figure 2. Diagnostic approach to hypokalemia (serum potassium [K^+] level of <3.5 mEq/L). A low serum K^+ level is identified. A high white blood cell count (WBC) can cause pseudohypokalemia.
DKA: diabetic ketoacidosis; GI: gastrointestinal; HTN: hypertension; NL: within normal limits; RTA: renal tubular acidosis; S_x: syndrome.
Serum K^+ is 0.5–0.9 mmol/L higher than plasma K^+.
Reproduced with permission of The McGraw-Hill Companies from *Harrison's Principles of Internal Medicine*, Twelfth Edition. Wilson JD, Braunwald E, Isselbacher KJ et al, editors. Copyright 2004, McGraw-Hill, Inc.

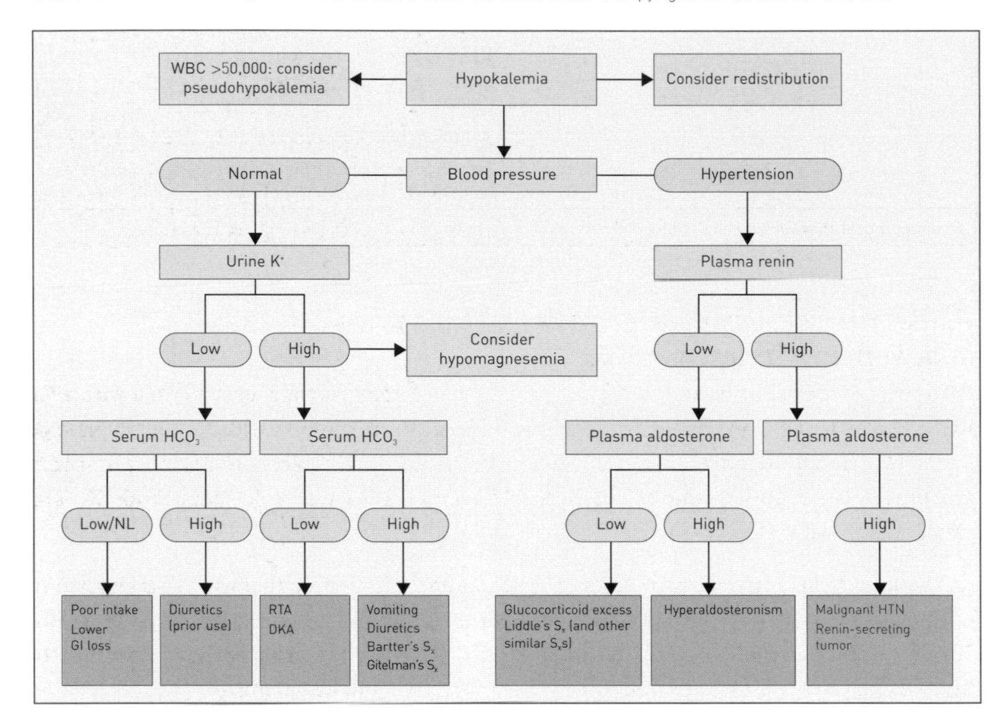

Diagnostic approach

Flow charts such as that shown in **Figure 2** are useful for determining the causes of hypokalemia. These, combined with a review of the causes of hypokalemia, will allow accurate diagnosis and provide a rational basis for treatment.

Treatment

General considerations

KCl supplementation – oral or intravenous – is the usual treatment for hypokalemia. The intravenous route is utilized when the patient cannot tolerate oral intake or in the case of more severe hypokalemia. Potassium repletion must be monitored carefully to achieve the goal of normokalemia (serum K^+ level of 4.0 mmol/L), and to avoid over-correction to hyperkalemia, which can be life-threatening. It is important to remember that there is a non-linear relationship between serum K^+ and TBK. A decrease in plasma K^+ levels from 4 mEq/L to 3 mEq/L represents a 100–200 mEq decline in TBK. Below 3 mEq/L, every 1 mEq/L fall in plasma K^+ reflects a 200–400 mEq decline in TBK [1,12]. It is important to include ongoing K^+ losses and maintenance requirements in the replacement prescription.

Table 5. Treatment of hypokalemia.

IV: intravenous; NPO: nil by mouth.

Indications for IV potassium replacement	Cardiac arrhythmia, rhabdomyolysis, paralysis, NPO Plasma [K^+]<2.0 mEq/L
IV administration	5–10 mEq/h can be given without cardiac monitoring in a stable patient 20 mEq/h requires cardiac monitoring and careful monitoring of serum K^+ When plasma K^+ ≥2.5 mEq/L, reduce infusion to 10 mEq/h IV KCl≤30–40 mEq/L concentration in a peripheral vein Maximum K^+ concentration 40 mEq/L in a peripheral vein and 60 mEq/L in a central vein
Change to oral therapy when feasible	High [K^+] foods. Follow serum K^+ closely

Guidelines for oral potassium replacement in patients with hypokalemia

Alkalosis or normal acid–base status in patients with hypokalemia is best treated with KCl. KCl can also be used in patients with acidosis, but supplementation with K^+ bicarbonate or K^+ citrate has the added benefit of co-administering alkali. K^+ gluconate and K^+ phosphate are further alternatives, with K^+ phosphate having a particular role when both K^+ and phosphorous deficiency are present [12].

KCl replacement is necessary in 10%–15% of patients on diuretic therapy. Maintenance of normokalemia is achieved by giving a higher dose of KCl (40–100 mEq daily as opposed to 30–50 mEq per day). A dose of KCl of 20 mEq daily is usually sufficient for prevention of hypokalemia in patients on diuretics. Target serum K^+ should be 4.0 mEq/L [12].

Guidelines for intravenous potassium replacement in patients with hypokalemia

Patients unable to tolerate fluids or enteral nutrition, those with excessive losses, or those with profound hypokalemia (<2 mEq/L) will require intravenous K^+ replacement (see **Table 5**). Cardiac arrhythmias, rhabdomyolysis, paralysis, nil by mouth status, and plasma K^+ levels of <3.0 mEq/L in the high-risk patient all suggest a need for intravenous K^+. Neuromuscular weakness syndromes due to hypokalemia can impair ventilator weaning and aggravate metabolic alkalosis and hepatic encephalopathy. In a hemodynamically stable patient without cardiac arrhythmias, KCl can be given at 5–10 mEq/h without cardiac monitoring. KCl at 20 mEq/h (in stable or unstable patients), however, requires cardiac monitoring and careful monitoring of serum K^+. When plasma K^+ levels are >3 mEq/L, the infusion rate should be reduced to 10 mEq/h. Monitoring serum K^+ is necessary every 1–4 hours initially to assure appropriate correction and to avoid life-threatening hyperkalemia [12,15].

Care should be taken in the administration of K^+ supplementation in patients on ACE inhibitors, angiotensin receptor blockers (ARBs), and spironolactone, and especially in patients with underlying kidney disease. Usual practice in patients with CKD placed on ACE

Table 6. Causes of hyperkalemia.

Reproduced from *Primer on Kidney Diseases*, Second Edition, Allon M. Chapter 13: Disorders of potassium metabolism:98–106. Copyright 2004, with permission from Elsevier.

Pseudohyperkalemia	Hemolysis Thrombocytosis Severe leukocytosis Fist clenching
Abnormal potassium distribution	Insulin deficiency β-Blockers Metabolic or respiratory acidosis Familial hyperkalemic periodic paralysis
Abnormal potassium release from cells	Rhabdomyolysis Tumor lysis syndrome
Decreased renal excretion	Acute or chronic kidney disease Aldosterone deficiency (eg, type IV renal tubular acidosis). Frequently associated with diabetic nephropathy, chronic interstitial nephritis, or obstructive nephropathy Adrenal insufficiency (Addison's disease) Drugs that inhibit potassium excretion Kidney diseases that impair distal tubule function: - sickle cell anemia - systemic lupus erythematosus

inhibitors or ARBs is to obtain measurements of blood urea nitrogen, serum creatinine, and electrolytes 5–7 days after beginning therapy with these medications.

A common intensive case unit practice is to give 10–20 mEq of KCl intravenously in 100 mL of normal saline over 1 hour as K^+ supplementation in patients with profound hypokalemia or cardiac arrhythmias: 20 mEq KCl leads to an average increase in serum K^+ of 0.25 mmol/L when administered in this manner. Serum K^+ should be monitored 1 hour post dose, and continuous cardiac monitoring should be performed. A change to oral therapy when feasible is recommended [12,15].

Hyperkalemia

Definition

Hyperkalemia is defined as a serum K^+ level of >5.5 mEq/L, and usually becomes symptomatic when serum K^+ is >6 mEq/L [1,8]. However, in over 50% of patients with CKD, normal serum K^+ may be >5.0 mEq/L as the patients have adapted to this level [16]. In such circumstances, the definition of hyperkalemia changes.

Demography

Hyperkalemia has a reported incidence of 1.1%–10% in hospitalized patients. The 1993 United States Renal Disease System (USRDS) database of patients with end-stage renal disease (ESRD) reported that hyperkalemia was responsible for 1.9% of deaths. However,

Table 7. Common medications causing hyperkalemia: "iatrogenesis fulminans".

ACE: angiotensin-converting enzyme; NSAIDs: nonsteroidal anti-inflammatory drugs.

Reprinted from *The American Journal of Medicine*, Volume 109, Perazella MA, Drug-induced hyperkalemia: old culprits and new offenders:307–14. Copyright 2004, with permission from Excerpta Medica.

Medication	Reported percentage of patients who develop hyperkalemia from the drug
Potassium supplements	3–24
β-Blockers	1–5
Digoxin	2–15
Potassium-sparing drugs	2–19
NSAIDs	10–46
ACE inhibitors	10–38
Angiotensin-II blockers	2–7
Trimethoprim	6–21
Pentamidine	5–24
Cyclosporine	11–44
Tacrolimus	15–53
Heparin	8–17

in a recently reported group of hospitalized patients with a serum K^+ level of >6 mmol/L, no patient died or experienced life-threatening arrhythmias, and only 14% exhibited electrocardiographic abnormalities consistent with hyperkalemia. The major causes of hyperkalemia in this series were renal failure, medications, and hyperglycemia [1,8,17].

Etiologies

Possible etiologies of hyperkalemia are listed in **Table 6**. Pseudohyperkalemia due to test tube cell lysis, thrombocytosis, or leukocytosis needs to be recognized. True hyperkalemia can be due to decreased renal excretion, transcellular shifts, high intake, or increased cellular release. Multiple drugs are associated with hyperkalemia (**Table 7**). Schepkens recently described life-threatening hyperkalemia in patients with mild CKD and cardiac disease who were prescribed ACE inhibitors and spironolactone [11]. Unusual sources of high K^+ intake need to be looked for, especially in patients with underlying kidney disease. These include herbal remedies and food supplements [1,8,17].

Physiological consequences

The signs and symptoms of hyperkalemia are similar to those of hypokalemia – predominantly neuromuscular weakness and cardiac arrhythmias – and are of major concern. Neuromuscular symptoms include weakness, paresthesias, and rarely paralysis, confusion, nausea, and vomiting. Hormonal changes include increased secretion of aldosterone and insulin.

Figure 3. Diagnostic approach to the hyperkalemic (serum potassium [K^+] level >5.5 mEq/L) patient.
ARF: acute renal failure; CKD: chronic kidney disease; IV: intravenous.
Reproduced with permission of The McGraw-Hill Companies from Schultze RG, Nissenson AR. Potassium: physiology and pathophysiology. In: *Clinical Disorders of Fluid and Electrolyte Metabolism*. Maxwell M, Kleeman C, editors. Copyright 2004, McGraw-Hill, Inc.

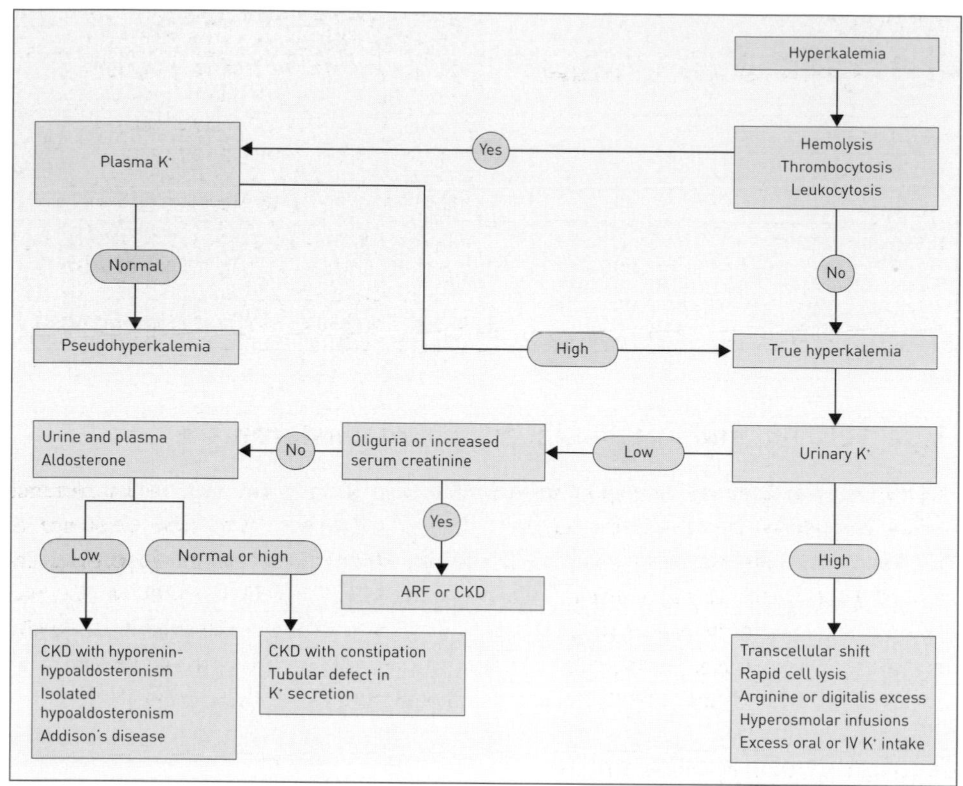

Renal consequences of hyperkalemia include natriuresis and decreased ammonia production. In patients with ESRD on dialysis, presentation with complaints of weakness and paresthesias always warrants a check of serum K^+. The presence of electrocardiographic abnormalities with hyperkalemia always warrants emergent treatment [17,18].

Diagnostic approaches

The diagnostic approach to hyperkalemia is illustrated in **Figure 3**. After an initial serum K^+ reading is obtained and pseudohyperkalemia is ruled out, urinary K^+ is then measured. Depending on the level of urinary K^+, further categorization of hyperkalemia is done. If the patient is oliguric and serum creatinine is elevated, acute or chronic kidney disease is the diagnosis. If the patient is not oliguric, the patient either has hypoaldosteronism or CKD (stage III or greater) with a predisposing condition for hyperkalemia, such as constipation, excessive K^+ intake, or an isolated tubular defect of K^+ secretion. If urinary K^+ is high, the possibility of transcellular shifts of K^+, cell lysis, or hyperosmolar infusions needs to be investigated. Potassium intake in excess of the ability to secrete a K^+ load is also a possibility.

Table 8. Acute treatment of hyperkalemia: remember "ACE".

ECF: extracellular fluid; ICF: intracellular fluid, IV: intravenous.
[a]Insulin, glucose, and albuteral potassium-lowering effects are additive but short term. Longer-term effects of $NaHCO_3$ and kayexalate are complementary.

A: Antagonism	IV calcium chloride or calcium gluconate: 10%, or 10 mL IV over 2–3 min. Can repeat in 5–10 min
C: Cellular redistribution: initiate ECF to ICF shifts[a]	Insulin and glucose: 50 g of 50% dextrose (1 Amp), and 5–10 units of regular insulin IV: onset 15 min
	β_2-adrenergic agonists, eg, albuterol nebulized @ 20 mg over 20 min: onset 30 min
	$NaHCO_3$: 50 mEq (1 Amp) IV or 5% dextrose with 3 Amps providing 150 mEq/L as an infusion: onset 3–4 h
E: Excretion	Kayexalate: 25–50 g in 100–200 mL 20% sorbitol orally or as a retention enema: onset 1–2 h, duration 4–6 h
	Diuretics: furosemide IV
	Dialysis: hemodialysis preferred for rapid correction

Hyperkalemia and hyporeninemic hypoaldosteronism

Patients with a diagnosis of hyporenin–hypoaldosteronism present with hyperchloremic metabolic acidosis, hyperkalemia, and mild renal insufficiency (creatinine clearance of 30–50 mL/min). This is often seen in patients with diabetes mellitus in whom hyperglycemia-induced hyperosmolality and insulin deficiency cause ICF to ECF shifts of K^+, and hypoaldosteronism decreases renal excretion of K^+. Drugs such as ACE inhibitors, ARBs, and spironolactone can mimic this effect and cause hyporenin–hypoaldosteronism. Treatment includes withdrawal of offending drugs or mineralocorticoid therapy [8,9].

Treatment of hyperkalemia

General considerations in the treatment of hyperkalemia include elimination of exogenous K^+ administration, discontinuance of drugs predisposing to hyperkalemia, a search for unusual sources of K^+ intake, electrocardiographic monitoring, and careful follow-up of serum K^+ post treatment (see **Table 6**). Treatment of acute hyperkalemia is outlined in **Table 8**. Essentially, this involves antagonism of the arrhythmogenic effects of hyperkalemia with calcium; cellular redistribution of K^+ from the ECF to the ICF with insulin and glucose, albuterol, and sodium bicarbonate; and promoting the excretion of K^+ using the ion exchange resin kayexalate (sodium polystyrene sulfonate), diuretics to increase renal excretion if feasible, and hemodialysis if necessary. It should be remembered that calcium antagonizes the effects of K^+ but does not remove K^+. Likewise, insulin and glucose, albuterol, and sodium bicarbonate shift K^+ from ECF to the ICF but do not lead to a net loss of K^+. Over a period of time the K^+ will return to the ECF, reproducing hyperkalemia. In selected situations, repeat treatment with insulin and dextrose or a continuous insulin infusion with 10% dextrose in water and with careful follow-up of blood glucose and serum K^+ may be necessary. The mnemonic "ACE" (antagonism, cellular redistribution, excretion) can be helpful in remembering the treatment for hyperkalemia. If hyperkalemia is refractory to treatment then hemodialysis or continuous renal replacement will be necessary (see **Section 4**) [1,8,10,17].

Mineralocorticoids may be useful in the chronic treatment of hyporenin–hypoaldosteronism. Addison's disease requires replacement of glucocorticoids and mineralocorticoids. A low K^+ diet (2 g K^+) may be necessary for long-term treatment.

References

1. Linas SL, Kellerman PS. Disorders of Potassium Metabolism. In: Feehally J, Johnson RJ, editors. *Comprehensive Clinical Nephrology*. St Louis, MI: Mosby, 2000.
2. Field M, Berliner R, Giebisch G. Renal Regulation of Potassium Balance. In: Narins RG, editor. *Clinical Disorders of Fluid and Electrolyte Metabolism*. 5th ed. New York, NY: McGraw-Hill Health Professions Division, 1993:147–74.
3. Stanton BA, Koeppen, BM. Renal System. In: Berne RM, Levy MN, editors. *Physiology*. St Louis, MI: Mosby, 1993.
4. Sterns RH, Cox M, Feig PU et al. Internal potassium balance and the control of the plasma potassium concentration. *Medicine (Baltimore)* 1981;60:339–54.
5. Gennari FJ. Hypokalemia. *N Engl J Med* 1998;339:451–8.
6. Adrogue HJ, Madias NE. Changes in plasma potassium concentration during acute acid–base disturbances. *Am J Med* 1981;71:456–67.
7. Weiner ID, Wingo CS. Hypokalemia-consequences, causes, and correction. *J Am Soc Nephrol* 1997;8:1179–88.
8. Allon M. Disorders of Potassium Metabolism. In: Greenburg A, editor. *Primer on Kidney Diseases*. 2nd ed. New York, NY: National Kidney Foundation, 1998:98–105.
9. Perazella MA. Drug-induced hyperkalemia: old culprits and new offenders. *Am J Med* 2000;109:307–14.
10. Allon M. Treatment and prevention of hyperkalemia in end-stage renal disease. *Kidney Int* 1993;43:1197–209.
11. Schepkens H, Vanholder R, Billiouw JM et al. Life-threatening hyperkalemia during combined therapy with angiotensin-converting enzyme inhibitors and spironolactone: an analysis of 25 cases. *Am J Med* 2001;110:438–41.
12. Cohn JN, Kowey PR, Whelton PK et al. New guidelines for potassium replacement in clinical practice: a contemporary review by the National Council on Potassium in Clinical Practice. *Arch Intern Med* 2000;160:2429–36.
13. Kurtz I. Molecular pathogenesis of Bartter's and Gitelman's syndromes. *Kidney Int* 1998;54:1396–410.
14. Brater DC. Diuretic therapy. *N Engl J Med* 1998;339:387–95.
15. Kruse JA, Carlson RW. Rapid correction of hypokalemia using concentrated intravenous potassium chloride infusions. *Arch Intern Med* 1990;150:613–7.
16. Gennari FJ, Segal AS. Hyperkalemia: An adaptive response in chronic renal insufficiency. *Kidney Int* 2002;62:1–9.
17. Acker CG, Johnson JP, Palevsky PM et al. Hyperkalemia in hospitalized patients: causes, adequacy of treatment, and results of an attempt to improve physician compliance with published therapy guidelines. *Arch Intern Med* 1998;158:917–24.
18. Gabow P, Peterson L. Disorders of Potassium Metabolism. In: Schrier R, editor. *Renal and Electrolyte Disorders.* 2nd ed. New York, NY: Little Brown and Company, 1980.

Part 5: Calcium, magnesium, and phosphorus

Richard N Hellman

Calcium

Calcium metabolism

Only 0.1% of total body calcium is found in the extracellular fluid (ECF), with 99% of total body calcium in bone mineral. Cell cytosolic calcium is one thousandth (0.001) of the ECF calcium concentration or 100 nmol/L. Serum calcium is 40% protein bound, mostly to albumin, 10% is complexed to phosphate, citrate, and carbonate, and 50% is ionized. Ionized and complexed calcium are filtered by the kidney. A fall in serum albumin of 1 g/dL from a normal of 4 g/dL is associated with a 0.8 mg/dL (0.20 mmol/L) fall in total serum calcium. Therefore, one must know the serum albumin concentration to interpret the serum calcium volume. For example, if the serum albumin is 2.0 g/dL and calcium is 9.5 mg/dL, then hypercalcemia exists. A fall of 0.1 pH units will cause a rise of approximately 0.1 mEq/L in ionized calcium as increased hydrogen ion concentrations displace calcium from albumin.

The average daily American diet contains 800 mg (20 mmol) of calcium, with a net absorption of 160 mg (4 mmol) (20% absorption rate/day). Increased 1,25-dihydroxy-vitamin D_3 (1,25$(OH)_2D_3$) is the principal hormonal regulator of intestinal calcium absorption. Binders of calcium, such as oxalate or phosphate, can reduce intestinal absorption of calcium. Oral medications such as prednisone also reduce calcium absorption.

The kidney reabsorbs 98% of the filtered load of calcium, with a calcium excretion rate of about 4 mmol/day, equal to net intestinal absorption. About 65% of the filtered load of calcium is reabsorbed in the proximal tubule via a mechanism linked to sodium reabsorption, 25% in the loop of Henle, and 8%–10% in the distal convoluted tubule. The distal convoluted tubule is the major regulator of urinary calcium excretion.

Distal convoluted tubule calcium reabsorption is increased by parathyroid hormone (PTH), phosphate depletion, and hydrochlorothiazide diuretic, and decreased by metabolic acidosis and increased aldosterone levels.

Serum calcium varies by <10% and is maintained at a level between 9.0 mg/dL and 10.4 mg/dL (2.25–2.6 mmol/L) if serum albumin is normal. The maintenance of normocalcemia is accomplished by a complex interaction between intestine, bone, and kidney through the interaction of PTH and 1,25$(OH)_2D_3$. PTH stimulates calcium reabsorption and phosphorus excretion in the distal convoluted tubule, stimulates bone mineral turnover, and increases the serum level of 1,25$(OH)_2D_3$, facilitating intestinal calcium absorption. PTH secretion is stimulated by decreased ionized serum calcium and hyperphosphatemia, and is inhibited by 1,25$(OH)_2D_3$ and hypomagnesemia [1].

Table 1. Differential diagnosis of hypercalcemia.

ATN: acute tubular necrosis; ESRD: end-stage renal disease; HPTH: hyperparathyroidism; MEN: multiple endocrine neoplasia: PTH: parathyroid hormone; PTHrP: parathyroid hormone-related protein.

Increased PTH: primary HPTH	MEN Lithium
Increased gut absorption	Milk-alkaline syndrome Vitamin D mediated Vitamin D toxicosis Granulomatous disease
Increased renal reabsorption	Thiazide diuretics Primary HPTH Post renal transplant
Increased bone resorption	Humoral hypercalcemia malignancy (PTHrP) Bone lytic lesions/tumor invasion Immobilization Thyrotoxicosis
Miscellaneous	Vitamin D intoxication Benign familial hypercalcemia Diuretic phase of myoglobinuric ATN ESRD with adynamic bone disease and calcium and/or vitamin D therapy Aluminum associated osteomalasia Vitamin A intoxication Pheochromocytoma Adrenal insufficiency

Acute hypercalcemia

Definition

Hypercalcemia is defined as an increase in the concentration of ionized serum calcium. A serum calcium of >10.5 mg/dL (2.60 mmol/L) and a normal serum albumin indicates hypercalcemia. Severe hypercalcemia is defined as >14 mg/dL (3.5 mmol/L), a level usually associated with symptoms requiring emergent treatment. An ionized serum calcium should be obtained if there is any question about the validity of total serum calcium [2]. Thrombocytosis with platelet counts of >700,000/mm^3 can falsely elevate serum calcium due to secretion of calcium from activated platelets [3]. When serum calcium is moderately increased to 12–14 mg/dL (3.0–3.5 mmol/L), the clinical manifestations serve as a guide to the type and necessity of therapy [2].

Clinical presentation

Clinical manifestations of hypercalcemia are evidenced by gastrointestinal, cardiovascular, renal, and central nervous system (CNS) findings. Gastrointestinal manifestations include anorexia, nausea, vomiting, constipation, and acute pancreatitis. Cardiovascular manifestations include hypertension and a shortened QT interval, and increased digitalis sensitivity. Renal manifestations include polyuria due to nephrogenic diabetes insipidus, polydipsia, and nephrocalcinosis. CNS symptoms and signs include apathy, altered cognition, drowsiness, obtundation, and coma.

Table 2. Blood tests for diagnosing hypercalcemia.

FBH: familial benign hypercalcemia; HPTH: hyperparathyroidism; P: serum phosphorus level; PTH: parathyroid hormone level; PTHrP: parathyroid hormone-related protein level; SPEP: Serum protein electrophoresis; TSH: thyroid-stimulating hormone level.

Primary HPTH	Elevated Ca^{2+}, low or normal P, elevated intact PTH
Cancer (majority: humoral)	Elevated Ca^{2+}, low or normal P, suppressed PTH, elevated PTHrP
Cancer (minority: bone metastases)	Elevated Ca^{2+}, suppressed intact PTH and PTHrP
Lymphoma (rare)	Elevated Ca^{2+}, P, and $1{,}25(OH)_2D_3$, suppressed PTH and PTHrP
Myeloma	Anemia, elevated Ca^{2+}, suppressed PTH, low PTHrP (most cases), monoclonal spike in SPEP
Thyrotoxicosis	Elevated Ca^{2+}, high normal P, suppressed PTH and TSH, elevated T4 and/or T3
Granulomatous disease	Elevated Ca^{2+}, P, and $1{,}25(OH)_2D_3$, suppressed PTH and PTHrP
FBH	Elevated Ca^{2+}, elevated or normal Mg^{2+}, low or normal P, inappropriately normal (85%) or slightly elevated (15%) PTH
Vitamin D toxicity	Elevated Ca^{2+}, P, and $1{,}25(OH)_2D_3$, suppressed PTH and PTHrP
Lithium	Elevated Ca^{2+} and intact PTH

Table 3. Other tests for diagnosing for hypercalcemia.

ACE: angiotensin-converting enzyme; FBH: familial benign hypercalcemia; HPTH: hyperparathyroidism; MEN: multiple endocrine neoplasia; *RET*: rearranged during transfection.

Urine tests	Specific diagnostic tests
Cancer and primary HPTH: elevated Ca^{2+} excretion	Skeletal lesions and bone marrow plasmacytosis in myeloma
Myeloma: Bence-Jones protein or M-spike	Elevated ACE levels in sarcoidosis
FBH: reduced Ca^{2+} excretion (<100 mg/day); Ca^{2+}/creatinine clearance (<0.01)	Mutations in *RET* proto-oncogene in MEN2
Vitamin D toxicity, granulomatous disease: marked hypercalciuria	

There is a great variability of symptoms for any given level of serum calcium due to patient age, volume status, acuity of hypercalcemia, and concomitant medical conditions. Symptoms may have alternative etiologies in borderline hypercalcemia. If serum calcium is >14 mg/dL (3.5 mmol/L), the symptoms are most likely to be hypercalcemia-related [2]. Bone pain may be present with osseous metastases or multiple myeloma. Cough, dyspnea, and lymphadenopathy may signal hypercalcemia due to granulomatous disease.

Mechanisms of hypercalcemia

Accelerated bone resorption caused by osteoclast activation by PTH or parathyroid hormone-related protein (PTHrP), cytokines, and tumoral calcitriol production may be mechanisms of hypercalcemia.

Demography

Hypercalcemic crisis (serum calcium >14 mg/dL) is usually due to underlying malignancy (70%), or primary hyperparathyroidism (20%). Hypercalcemia occurs in 10%–20% of cancer patients, most commonly due to lung cancer, breast cancer, and multiple myeloma. The prognosis for tumor-related hypercalcemia is poor [4].

Table 4. Medical treatments for hypercalcemia.

CHF: congestive heart failure; CNS: central nervous system; IM: intramuscular; IV: intravenous; SC: subcutaneous.

Calcitonin	(IM or SC) 4–8 IU/kg every 12 h Effective in 4–6 h in 60%–70% of patients Tachyphylaxis may occur in 2–3 days
Bisphosphonates	Pamidronate: 60–90 mg IV every 1–4 weeks. If serum Ca^{2+} is <12 mg/dL, give 30 mg, if 12–13.5 mg/dL give 60 mg, if >13.5 mg/dL, give 90 mg. Can repeat in 7 days Etridonate: (7.5 mg/kg IV) over 4 h, daily for 3–7 days. Reduce dose by 50% in renal failure Zoledronic acid: 1–4 mg, effects last 32–43 days
Mithramycin	25 mg/kg IV over 4–6 h (rarely used)
Gallium nitrate	Rarely used
Dialysis	If renal failure, CHF, and/or CNS findings Use of low or zero calcium bath

Differential diagnosis

The differential diagnosis for hypercalcemia is seen in **Table 1**, and useful tests for making a diagnosis are listed in **Tables 2** and **3**. Initial laboratory testing should include blood urea nitrogen (BUN), creatinine, electrolytes, total and ionized calcium, phosphorus, serum albumin, magnesium, alkaline phosphatase, PTH, complete blood count, an electrocardiogram, and possibly PTHrP if neoplasm is suspected. PTH levels are high in hyperparathyroidism and low in malignancy. Malignancy is usually clinically apparent. Common neoplasms associated with hypercalcemia are lung, breast, and renal cell carcinoma, multiple myeloma, and, rarely, non-Hodgkin lymphoma. Parathyroid-related protein is elevated in malignancy. Familial hypocalciuric hypercalcemia is an inherited defect in the calcium sensor of the parathyroid cells. It is often confused with primary hyperparathyroidism. This is not a disease state, and parathyroidectomy is contraindicated [4].

Treatment

The first step in the treatment of hypercalcemia is to assess severity. Symptomatic hypercalcemia, with calcium levels of >12–14 mg/dL (3.00–3.50 mmol/L) with a normal serum albumin, warrants treatment, but serum calcium levels of above the upper limit of normal or elevated with symptomatic hypercalcemia may require more aggressive therapy. After assessing severity, the next step should be assessment of volume status, urine output, and cardiovascular status. Volume depletion is common in hypercalcemia related to nephrogenic diabetes insipidus and polyuria. The initial goals of treatment are to increase urinary calcium excretion with isotonic saline volume expansion and loop diuretics following appropriate volume expansion, and to decrease bone reabsorption with calcitonin and bisphosphonates. Volume expansion and the use of loop diuretics may be all that is required to normalize serum calcium in less severe hypercalcemia. In special cases of increased calcium absorption (due to increased intake, vitamin D intoxication, vitamin A intoxication, and/or hematologic malignancy) corticosteroid treatment is indicated (see **Table 4**).

Etiology-specific therapy includes parathyroidectomy, specific cancer treatment (surgery, radiation therapy, or chemotherapy), prednisone in the treatment of granulomatous disease, and treatment of hyperthyroidism with β-blockade and specific anti-thyroid therapy.

Table 5. Clinical presentations of hypocalcemia.

CHF: congestive heart failure; ECG: electrocardiogram.

Reproduced with permission from Zabya GP, Chernow B. Hypocalcemia in critical illness. *JAMA* 1986;256:1924–9.

Neurologic	Cardiovascular	Respiratory	Psychiatric
Chvostek's and Trousseau's signs	Arrhythmia	Apnea	Anxiety
Muscle cramps and spasms	CHF	Bronchospasm	Depression
Weakness	Hypotension	Laryngeal spasm	Dementia
Paresthesia	ECG abnormalities of QT and ST interval prolongation. T wave inversion		Psychosis
Seizure			Irritability

In the presence of renal failure, congestive heart failure, and neurologic symptoms, acute hemodialysis with a zero or low calcium bath or continuous venovenous hemofiltration may be necessary. Calcitonin is contraindicated in patients allergic to salmon and may be associated with pruritus, nausea, vomiting, and dizziness. Calcitonin does have a rapid onset of action, but is a weak hypocalcemic agent with a maximum reduction of serum calcium of 1–2 mg/dL. Tachyphylaxis can also occur. Pamidronate can cause leukopenia, fever, arthralgia, and myalgia. It is contraindicated in patients with severe renal failure and hypersensitivity to the drug, and is also contraindicated in pregnancy. Mithramycin and galium are now rarely used in the acute treatment of hypercalcemia, and are associated with significant renal and bone marrow toxicities [2]. The follow-up for hypercalcemia treatment should include assessment of intake and output (I and O), daily weight, hemodynamics, and CNS and cardiac status. Frequent monitoring of serum calcium, phosphorus, magnesium, electrolytes, BUN, and creatinine are necessary.

Acute hypocalcemia

Definition

Hypocalcemia is defined as a reduction in serum ionized calcium. In general, this occurs as a result of decreased levels or function of PTH or vitamin D, cellular shifts, magnesium deficiency, and chelation effects as occur in sepsis and blood transfusions with citrated blood [1].

Demography

The majority of patients (80%) in medical or surgical intensive care units (ICUs) are hypocalcemic as measured by total serum calcium level. Between 15% and 40% of patients have serum ionized calcium levels <1 mmol/L (4 mg/dL). Twenty percent of all patients undergoing cardiopulmonary bypass surgery and 30%–40% of patients with multiple trauma have serum ionized calcium levels of 0.8–1 mmol/L. Symptomatic ionized hypocalcemia occurs at levels <0.7 mmol/L, and life threatening complications occur when ionized calcium is <0.5 mmol/L (2 mg/dL) [5–7].

Clinical presentation

Hypocalcemia in the ICU often presents as an isolated laboratory finding but can be associated with multisystem findings involving the neuropsychiatric, respiratory, and cardiovascular systems (see **Table 5**) [6].

Table 6. Differential diagnosis of hypocalcemia.

IV: intravenous.

Hypoparathyroidism	Post surgical Post radiation therapy Congenital Autoimmune
Vitamin D deficiency	Renal failure Poor nutrition Malabsorption Short bowel Cirrhosis
Pancreatitis	
Hypomagnesemia	
Rhabdomyolysis	
Hungry bone syndrome	
Tumor lysis	
Hyperphosphatemia	
Sepsis	
Toxic shock syndrome	
Acute respiratory alkalosis	
Metabolic alkalosis	
Chelation	Citrated blood Albumin IV contrast
Fat embolism	
Pseudohypoparathyroidism	

Diagnosis

A low total serum calcium level should prompt the measurement of a serum ionized calcium level to confirm hypocalcemia, and the differential diagnosis should then be reviewed (see **Table 6**). Useful diagnostic tests include serum phosphorus, PTH, and vitamin D levels.

Hypoparathyroidism is characterized by hypocalcemia, a high or normal serum phosphorus level, and a low PTH level. Hypocalcemia due to magnesium deficiency is usually characterized by hypomagnesemia, a normal serum phosphorus level, and a low PTH level due to magnesium suppression of PTH secretion, but can present with normal serum magnesium in the setting of hypocalcemia, hypokalemia, an abnormal magnesium tolerance test and tetany, seizures, and arrhythmias. Empiric repletion of magnesium in these circumstances may be indicated if renal function is normal. Vitamin D deficiency is characterized by low or normal serum phosphorus, an increased PTH level, a low vitamin D level, and reduced urinary calcium excretion. Urine testing in hypocalcemia includes measurement of calcium and creatinine.

Table 7. Hypocalcemia treatment: what to do first.

D5W: 5% dextrose in water; IV: intravenous.

Assess severity of symptoms
Assess integrity of airway
Parenteral Ca^{2+} salts for severe or life-threatening symptoms:
- Ca^{2+} gluconate (93 mg Ca^{2+}/10 mL)
- Infuse two ampules over 10–20 mins
- IV Ca^{2+} gluconate infusion: 60 mL in 500 mL D5W (1 mg/mL) infuse at 0.5–2.0 mg/kg/h to control symptoms
- Measure serum total and ionized Ca^{2+} every 4–6 h
- Treatment goal: maintain serum Ca^{2+} at 8–9 mg/dL or ionized Ca^{2+} approximately 1.0 mmol/L
- Begin oral Ca^{2+} supplements and vitamin D as soon as possible and discontinue IV calcium
- If Mg^{2+} depleted, replete with magnesium salts first
- WARNING: Ca^{2+} chloride – 273 mg Ca^{2+}/10 mL as opposed to 93 mg/10 mL in calcium gluconate

Table 8. Hypocalcemia treatment: general and specific measures.

CKD: chronic kidney disease.

General measures	Specific therapy
Treat symptoms, not just lab values: - Maintain serum Ca^{2+} 8.5–9.0 mg/dL ionized serum Ca^{2+} approximately 1.0 mmol/L - Maintain urine Ca^{2+}≤300 mg/day	Oral Ca^{2+}, supplements Add vitamin D metabolites depending on severity and titrate: - Ergocalciferol - Calcitriol if CKD Thiazide diuretics as adjunctive therapy to increase renal Ca^{2+} reabsorption

Table 9. Regimens for oral calcium and vitamin D supplements.

DHT: dihydrotachysterol; USP: United States Pharmacopeia.

[a]GlaxoSmithKline, Pittsburgh, PA, USA. [b]Bone Care International, Middleton, WI, USA.

Oral calcium	Oral vitamin D
Calcium carbonate (Os-Cal[a], TUMS[a]): 250 mg/625 mg tablet; or 500 mg/1500 mg tablet.	Vitamin D_2 (ergocalciferol, calciferol): 50,000–400,000 U/day; 50,000 USP units/tablet)
TUMS[a] is available in 200 mg, 300 mg (ES), 400 mg (ultra), and 500 mg tablets	DHT: (0.125, 0.2, 0.4 mg tablets); dose 0.2–1 mg/day
Calcium citrate (Citrucel[a]): 200–250 mg/950 mg tablet is the most bioavailable, but avoid its use in chronic kidney disease due to citrate-enhanced gut aluminum absorption	25(OH)D_3 (calcifediol): 50–100 μg/day (20–50 μg capsules)
	1,25(OH)$_2D_3$ (calcitriol): 0.25–1 μg/day (0.25 and 0.5 μg tablets)
	Doxercalciferol (Hectorol[b]): 2.5–10 μg; 3 × week (2.5 μg tablets)

Treatment

General considerations in the treatment of hypocalcemia are to treat the symptoms and not just the laboratory values; maintain serum calcium at the lower limit of normal (>8.0 mg/dL and <9.0 mg/dL, ionized calcium of 1 mmol/L); keep urinary calcium at <300 mg/day; and correct hypomagnesemia if present. Calcium repletion and vitamin D treatment are the mainstays of therapy. The use of thiazide diuretics to minimize hypercalciuria may be necessary. **Tables 7** and **8** provide details on hypocalcemia treatment. Oral therapy should be begun as soon as is feasible. Regimens for oral calcium therapy and vitamin D therapy are given in **Table 9**. Careful monitoring of hemodynamics, electrocardiogram, serum calcium, phosphorus, magnesium, BUN, serum creatinine, electrolytes, and urinary calcium are necessary in the follow-up of hypocalcemia treatment.

Magnesium

Magnesium metabolism

Magnesium is the second most abundant intracellular cation after potassium and the fourth most abundant cation in the human body. It plays an important role in cellular function. In adults, total body magnesium is ~24 g or 1,000 mmol, with 60% located in bone, 39% intracellular, and 1% extracellular. An average diet includes 280 mg/day of magnesium, of which 205 mg is excreted by the gut and 75 mg by the kidney. Fractional intestinal absorption of magnesium in the proximal jejunum and ileum ranges from 25%–60%. Eighty percent of the total plasma magnesium is filtered at the glomerulus. Renal tubular handling of magnesium differs from that of other cations in that 60%–70% is reabsorbed in the thick ascending limb of the loop of Henle, with 30% reabsorption in the proximal tubule and the remainder in the distal tubule and cortical collecting duct. There is no appreciable renal tubular magnesium secretion, and control of renal magnesium homeostasis involves changes in tubular reabsorption. Three to five percent of the filtered load of magnesium is excreted by the kidney [8].

Factors and hormones influencing urinary magnesium excretion are hypercalcemia, hypermagnesemia, ECF volume expansion, decreased PTH levels, and acidosis. Cellular shifts of magnesium can be important in hypomagnesemic states.

Hypermagnesemia

Definition

Serum magnesium normally ranges between 1.7–2.1 mg/dL (0.70–0.85 mmol/L or 1.4–1.7 mEq/L).

Demography

Hypermagnesemia is usually iatrogenic, occurring in patients with renal functional impairment ingesting large amounts of magnesium.

Clinical manifestations

The level of serum magnesium correlates with symptoms and signs (see **Table 10**). Patients with a serum magnesium level of <3.6 mg/dL (1.5 mmol/L) are usually not symptomatic. At levels of >4 mEq/L there is inhibition of neuromuscular transmission, and deep tendon reflexes are abolished.

Diagnosis

The causes and differential diagnosis of hypermagnesemia are listed in **Table 11**. The presence of renal insufficiency and excess magnesium intake, either orally, rectally, or intravenously, are most common. Magnesium intoxication in women treated with magnesium sulfate for toxemia of pregnancy can occur. A serum magnesium measurement is indicated in patients with neuromuscular weakness, cardiac arrhythmia, or those patients receiving total parenteral nutrition (TPN), enteral nutrition, or magnesium therapy.

Table 10. Signs and symptoms of hypermagnesemia.

Magnesium level	Signs and symptoms
>4 mEq/L	Inhibition of neuromuscular transmission Deep tendon reflexes are abolished
>7 mEq/L	Lethargy
5–10 mEq/L	Hypotension and prolongation of the PR and QT intervals as well as QRS duration
>10 mEq/L	Paralysis of voluntary muscles and respiratory failure
>15 mEq/L	Complete heart block or asystole

Table 11. Causes of hypermagnesemia.

Increased intake	Decreased renal excretion	Redistribution
Excessive oral, rectal, or parenteral intake of magnesium with normal renal function (rare)	Excessive intake of magnesium-containing drugs (antacids, laxatives), potassium-sparing diuretics, or lithium in patients with renal insufficiency	Pheochromocytoma Acidosis

Treatment

The treatment of hypermagnesemia should begin with discontinuance of magnesium administration. Symptomatic patients with hypermagnesemia should be treated initially with intravenous calcium infusion, as calcium is a direct antagonist of magnesium. One ampule of calcium gluconate provides 93 mg of elemental calcium in 10 mL, and 1–2 ampules can be given over 5–10 minutes.

In patients with normal renal function, volume expansion and loop diuretics can increase magnesium excretion. In the presence of renal failure or hypermagnesemia unresponsive to therapy, acute hemodialysis or continuous renal replacement therapy (CRRT) is indicated. Serum magnesium, calcium, phosphorus, BUN, creatinine, electrolytes, I and O, and hemodynamic status need careful follow-up during and after therapy.

Hypomagnesemia

Definition

Normal serum magnesium ranges between 1.7 and 2.1 mg/dL (0.70–0.85 mmol/L or 1.4–1.7 mEq/L). A low serum magnesium of <1.5 mg/dL indicates significant magnesium deficiency. Predictors of magnesium deficiency are a low urinary fractional excretion of magnesium and retention of more than 75% of an infused magnesium load. The magnesium loading test is unreliable in patients with renal dysfunction or in patients on medications that can alter urinary magnesium excretion.

Demography

Hypomagnesemia is a common problem in hospitalized patients, and is seen in 10% of general hospital admissions and up to 65% of patients hospitalized in an ICU. It is especially common in patients with acute pancreatitis (25%–30%) [8].

Table 12. Differential diagnosis of hypomagnesemia.

Redistribution from extracellular to intracellular fluids	Insulin administration post therapy of diabetic ketoacidosis Hungry bone syndrome post parathyroidectomy Catecholamine excess states such as alcohol withdrawal syndrome Acute pancreatitis Excessive lactation
Reduced intake	Starvation Alcoholism Prolonged postoperative state
Reduced absorption	Specific gastrointestinal magnesium malabsorption Generalized malabsorption syndrome Post extensive bowel resections Diffuse bowel disease or injury Chronic diarrhea Laxative abuse
Extrarenal factors which increase magnesuria	Drug-induced losses: diuretics, aminoglycosides, digoxin, cisplatinum amphotericin B, foscarnet, cyclosporine Hormone-induced magnesuria: aldosteronism, hypoparathyroidism, hyperthyroidism Ion or nutrient induced tubular losses: hypercalcemia, extracellular fluid volume expansion Miscellaneous causes: phosphate depletion syndrome, alcohol ingestion

Clinical presentation

Hypomagnesemia should be considered in the presence of neuromuscular weakness, cardiac arrhythmias, refractory hypokalemia or hypocalcemia, and in the presence of depletion syndromes.

Symptoms are similar to those seen with hypocalcemia. These include apathy, depression, delirium, seizures, weakness, myoclonus, tetany, and coma. A positive Chvostek's sign and, less commonly, Trousseau's sign, can be seen. Electrocardiographic abnormalities include premature ventricular contractions, ventricular tachycardia, ventricular fibrillation, and torsades de pointes.

Diagnosis

The differential diagnosis of hypomagnesemia includes redistribution of magnesium from ECF to intracellular fluid, reduced intake, reduced absorption, and extrarenal factors that increase renal magnesium excretion. The differential diagnoses are listed in **Table 12**.

Treatment

Hypomagnesemia is treated with magnesium repletion. Parenteral administration is indicated for symptomatic hypomagnesemia, hypokalemia, hypocalcemia, or replacement of magnesium in TPN (see **Table 13**). As in all fluid and electrolyte disorders, appreciation of ongoing losses, deficits, and maintenance requirements is necessary. Oral magnesium regimens are listed in **Table 14**.

Patients with mild asymptomatic hypomagnesemia can be treated with oral magnesium 10–30 mEq/day in divided doses. Mild symptomatic hypomagnesemia can be treated

Table 13. Intravenous treatment of hypomagnesemia.

[a]Symptomatic magnesium deficiency usually reflects a total magnesium deficit of 1–2 mEq/Kg of body weight.

Magnesium sulfate	Don't just order a "vial"	Treatment goals
1–2 g (8–16 mEq) over 10 min for emergencies	Magnesium sulfate-50%: 50 mg (4 mEq/mL)	Maintain serum magnesium levels above lower limit of normal
Less urgent, 12 g (1 mEq/kg)[a] over 24 h	Magnesium sulfate-25%: 25 mg (2 mEq/mL)	Switch to oral preparations as soon as possible or when patient is not symptomatic
Then: 4–6 g/day for 3–5 days	Magnesium sulfate-10%: 10 mg (1 mEq/mL)	

Table 14. Oral treatment of hypomagnesemia.

[a]Niche Pharmaceuticals, Roanoke, TX, USA; [b]Purdue Products LP, Stamford, CT, USA; [c]Premier Chemicals, Middleburg Hts, OH, USA; [d]Magonate Sport, Fenton, MO, USA.

Product	Mag-Tab SR[a]	Slow-Mag[b]	MagOx[c] 400	Magonate[d]
Form of magnesium	L-lactate dihydrate	Chloride	Oxide	Gluconate
Elemental Mg^{2+}/dose	84 mg	64 mg	241 mg	27 mg
mEq Mg^{2+}/dose	7 mEq	5.26 mEq	19.8 mEq	2.2 mEq
Solubility	Excellent	High	Extremely low	Moderate
Oral absorption	41.1%	19.68%	2.00%	19.25%
Bioavailable (bio.) mEq Mg^{2+}/dose	2.87 mEq	1.04 mEq	0.39 mEq	0.42 mEq
Dose needed to provide approx. 5.7 mEq bio. Mg^{2+}/day	2 tablets	5–6 tablets	14 tablets	13 tablets

with 30–60 mEq/day of oral magnesium in divided doses. Therapy should be adjusted to patient symptoms, serum magnesium level, or magnesium retention test results. In cases of hypocalcemia or hypokalemia related to hypomagnesemia, monitoring of serum calcium, phosphorus, and potassium with electrolytes is necessary. The addition of the potassium-sparing diuretics amiloride or triamterene can reduce urinary magnesium excretion by increasing magnesium reabsorption in the cortical collecting duct. Gastrointestinal side effects, notably diarrhea, are common with oral magnesium salt therapy.

Phosphorus

Phosphorus metabolism

Ninety percent of phosphorus is in the bone mineral, 10% is intracellular, and 1% is extracellular. A normal serum concentration ranges between 2.5 and 4.5 mg/dL (0.81–1.45 mmol/L). Thirty percent of phosphorus is inorganic and 70% is organic contained within phospholipids. Serum phosphorus levels may vary by as much as 50% every day [1].

The average phosphorus dietary intake is 800 1,850 mg/day (26–60 mmol/day), of which 25 mmol is absorbed. Phosphorus absorption is regulated by $1,25(OH)_2D_3$ levels with passive intestinal absorption in the jejunum and ileum. The daily filtered load of phosphorus is 200 mmol, with 85% of serum phosphorus being ultra-filterable. Urine phosphorus excretion

Table 15. Hyperphosphatemia-specific therapies.

[a]GlaxoSmithKline, Pittsburgh, PA, USA; [b]Nabi Biopharmaceuticals, Boca Raton, FL, USA; [c]Genzyme, Cambridge, MA, USA.

Indications	All hyperphosphatemia should be treated, but ability to treat is limited
Treatment options	
Acute hyperphosphatemia	Intravenous volume repletion with normal saline will enhance renal excretion, add 10 U insulin and one ampule D50 to enhance cellular uptake. Optimal removal is obtained with dialysis but this is limited due to intracellular location of phosphorus
Chronic hyperphosphatemia	Dietary restriction to 800 mg/day (although this diet is very difficult to maintain)
	Phosphate binders: – Calcium carbonate, 500 mg elemental calcium with each meal (TUMS[a], OsCal[a]) – Calcium acetate, 667 mg (169 elemental calcium) with each meal (Phos-lo[b]) – Sevelamer HCl (Renagel[c]), 400 or 800 mg with each meal
	Choice of binder is dependent on serum calcium level and tolerability of agent. Number of pills needs to be titrated to oral intake of phosphorus and serum levels
	For severe hyperphosphatemia, short-term administration (ideally <4 weeks) of aluminum hydroxide (alternagel 30–60 mL or alu-caps 3–6 capsules) with each meal may be necessary

is 25 mmol/day on average, yielding a filtration fraction of 12.5%. In the kidney, 85% of phosphorus absorption occurs in the proximal tubule. PTH is the major hormonal regulator of phosphorus excretion. Increased PTH levels are phosphaturic [1].

Hyperphosphatemia

Definition

Hyperphosphatemia is defined as a serum phosphorus level of >5 mg/dL in adults. Hemolysis of cells may falsely elevate serum phosphorus.

Demography

Hyperphosphatemia most commonly occurs in the ICU as a result of renal failure, rhabdomyolysis, or tumor lysis syndrome.

Clinical presentation

Hyperphosphatemia is usually asymptomatic unless hypocalcemia occurs due to precipitation of insoluble calcium phosphate complexes and decreased $1,25(OH)_2D_3$ synthesis; then the symptoms are those of hypocalcemia. Chronic hyperphosphatemia in renal failure is associated with vascular calcifications and increased mortality in end-stage renal disease patients.

Differential diagnosis

Hyperphosphatemia occurs almost exclusively with impaired renal function. Other causes are tumor lysis syndrome, rhabdomyolosis, vitamin D intoxication, phosphate-containing enemas, or increased renal reabsorption occurring with hypoparathyroidism, thyrotoxicosis, or acromegaly.

Treatment

Treatment approaches include reduction in phosphorus intake and phosphorus binders to minimize intestinal absorption. Volume repletion with normal saline will enhance renal

Table 16. Differential diagnosis of hypophosphatemia.

ATN: acute tubular necrosis; DKA: diabetes ketoacidosis; TPN: total parenteral nutrition.

Hypophosphatemia	Decreased intestinal absorption, increased urinary losses, and/or extracellular to intracellular shift. Severe hypophosphatemia is usually due to a combination of factors
Decreased intestinal absorption	Antacid abuse, malabsorption, chronic diarrhea, vitamin D deficiency, starvation, anorexia, alcoholism
Increased urinary losses	Primary hyperparathyroidism, postrenal transplant, extracellular fluid volume expansion, glucosuria (after treating DKA), post-obstructive or resolving ATN diuresis, acetazolamide, Fanconi's syndrome, X-linked and vitamin D-dependent rickets, oncogenic osteomalacia
Redistribution	Respiratory alkalosis, alcohol withdrawal, severe burns, TPN, recovery from malnutrition when inadequate phosphate is provided (post-feeding syndrome), leukemic blast crisis

excretion, and the addition of dextrose and insulin will enhance increased cellular uptake. Hemodialysis or CRRT may be necessary (see **Table 15**).

Moderate hypophosphatemia

Definition

Moderate hypophosphatemia is defined as a serum phosphorus between 1.0 and 2.0 mg/dL or the lower limit of normal (2.5–4.5 mg/dL [0.81–1.45 mmol/L]). Severe hypophosphatemia is defined as a serum phosphorus level of <1 mg/dL. Hypophosphatemia may not reflect reduced total body phosphorus, since only 1% of total body phosphorus is extracellular [1].

Demography

Hypophosphatemia is common in the hospitalized patient. Ten percent of hospitalized alcoholics, 3% of hospitalized patients, and up to 70% of ICU patients on TPN have hypophosphatemia. Renal transplant patients can develop hypophosphatemia, as can patients with gastrointestinal disorders such as chronic diarrhea or malabsorption [8].

Clinical presentation

Symptoms are usually present if serum phosphorus is <1 mg/dL. These include neuromuscular weakness, paresthesias, encephalopathy, seizures, coma, rhabdomyolysis, congestive heart failure and cardiomyopathy, hemolysis, thrombocytopenia, bleeding, white cell dysfunction, decreased glomerular filtration rate, renal tubular abnormalities, and insulin resistance. Chronically, osteomalacia and rickets can occur.

Diagnosis

Diagnosis is based on serum phosphorus, symptoms, history, trends in serum phosphorus values, and a low urine phosphorus (<100 mg/day). In the presence of phosphaturia and an elevated serum calcium, hyperparathyroidism should be considered. In the presence of glycosuria and renal tubular acidosis, a diagnosis of Fanconi's syndrome should be considered. The differential diagnosis of hypophosphatemia is summarized in **Table 16**.

Therapy

General considerations in therapy are 1) careful assessment of severity and symptoms, so as not to over treat hypophosphatemia due to cellular shifts; 2) avoidance of metastatic

Table 17. Specific therapy for hypophosphatemia.

Goal of therapy	To provide 1,000 mg (32 mM)/day of elemental phosphorus with max of 3,000 mg/day
Oral	Skimmed milk (1,000 mg/quart), whole milk (850 mg/quart), neutraphos K^+ capsules (250 mg/capsule; max dose 3 tablets every 6 h), neutraphos solution (128 mg/mL solution)
Intravenous	Potassium phosphate (3 mmol/mL of phosphate, 4.4 mEq/mL of K^+), Na^+ phosphate (3 mmol/mL of phosphate, 4.0 mEq/mL of Na^+). Do not exceed 2 mg phosphorus/kg body weight every 6 h to avoid metastatic calcification
In hyperalimentation	To avoid refeeding syndrome ensure 450 mg phosphorus for each 1,000 kcal infused

calcification due to high calcium–phosphorus product; and 3) treatment of severe symptomatic hypophosphatemia with intravenous therapy. Asymptomatic hypophosphatemia can be treated with oral agents. The potassium and sodium load needs to be considered in patients with renal failure and congestive heart failure (see **Table 17**). Complications of oral phosphate therapy include diarrhea, hyperphosphatemia, hypocalcemia, and hyperkalemia with potassium phosphate preparations. Careful follow-up of serum calcium, phosphorus, magnesium, electrolytes, renal function, and acid–base status are necessary during treatment.

References

1. Bushinsky D. Disorders of calcium and phosphorus homeostasis. In: Greenberg A, editor. *Primer on Kidney Diseases*. 3rd ed. New York, NY: National Kidney Foundation. 2001;107–15.
2. Bilezikian JP. Management of acute hypercalcemia. *N Engl J Med* 1992;326:1196–203.
3. Howard MR, Ashwell S, Bond LR et al. Artefactual serum hyperkalaemia and hypercalcaemia in essential thrombocythaemia. *J Clin Pathol* 2000;53:105–9.
4. Ziegler R. Hypercalcemic crisis. *J Am Soc Nephrol* 2001;12(Suppl. 17):S3–9.
5. Zaloga GP, Chernow B. Hypocalcemia in critical illncss. *JAMA* 1986;256:1924–9.
6. Zivin JR, Gooley T, Zager RA et al. Hypocalcemia: a pervasive metabolic abnormality in the critically ill. *Am J Kidney Dis* 2001;37:689–98.
7. Suleiman M, Zaloga GP. How and when to manage ionized hypocalcemia in critically ill patients. *J Crit Illn* 1993;3:372–90.
8. Drueke T, Lacour B. Disorders of calcium, phosphate, and magnesium metabolism. In: Johnson R, Feehally J, editors. *Comprehensive Clinical Nephrology*. New York, NY: Mosby. 2003:Sect. 3(17);11.1–11.16.

Part 6: Nutrition

Edward Sha

The utility of nutritional support in improving the survival of critically ill patients remains a matter of controversy. In the recent SUPPORT study [1], Borum and colleagues examined the effects of enteral or parenteral nutrition in 6,298 seriously ill patients. The results were mixed: coma patients who received nutritional support had improved outcomes, while patients with respiratory failure or multiple organ dysfunction syndrome (MODS) with sepsis, cirrhosis, and chronic obstructive pulmonary disease and who received nutritional support experienced worse outcomes. Nevertheless, the prevailing opinion is that critically ill patients benefit from nutrition when administered correctly.

Physiology

Table 1 lists the metabolic changes generally seen in critically ill patients and those with acute renal failure (ARF).

Critically ill patients have an increased metabolic rate and typically require 30 kcal/kg/day; this figure should be increased by 15%–30% for patients with sepsis, severe burns, and respiratory failure requiring mechanical ventilation. The etiology of this hypermetabolic state remains a point of investigation but has been associated with fever as well as circulating cytokines [2]. The energy expenditure for an average-sized, critically ill individual rarely exceeds 3,000 kcal/day even for patients with MODS. When ARF is present, the energy requirements should be based on the patient's other medical conditions since ARF does not necessarily increase or decrease the metabolic rate.

Critically ill patients also require a greater proportion of their energy requirements to be administered as protein, with a recommended range of 1.2–1.5 g/kg/day. Patients receiving renal replacement therapy (RRT), especially continuous RRT (CRRT), have additional protein losses and require greater protein supplementation. Two studies suggest that patients

Table 1. Metabolic changes seen in critically ill patients.

Increased protein catabolism
Impaired amino acid clearance
Glucose intolerance
Release of glucagons
Increased gluconeogenesis
Increased urea production
Unsuppressed lipid oxidation
Impaired lipolysis
Impaired lipid clearance
Release of cytokines

Table 2. Recommendations for the nutritional management of critically ill patients.

CRRT: continuous renal replacement therapy; TPN: total parenteral nutrition.

General	Enteral feeding	Parenteral feeding
Initiate early Prescribe caloric intake 30–40 kcal/kg/day Prescribe protein intake 1.5–2.0 g/kg/day	Preferred modality Use renal formulas (high protein, low volume)	Reduce Na^+ content by 50%–75% for oliguric patients Use chloride to balance the TPN solution Remove K^+, Ca^{2+}, and Mg^{2+} if patient on CRRT

on RRT should receive 1.8–2.0 g/kg/day of protein [3,4]. To ensure adequate nitrogen intake, the daily urea nitrogen content in waste fluids such as urine or dialysis effluent can be collected or calculated from several random samples to assess whether nitrogen intake matches nitrogen output [3,4].

Hyperglycemia is commonly seen in critically ill patients. In a landmark prospective study, van den Berghe and colleagues randomized critically ill patients to conventional insulin treatment or intensive insulin treatment using an insulin drip to maintain the blood sugar level between 80 and 100 mg/dL [5]. Overall mortality fell from 8.0% in the conventional treatment group to 4.6% in the intensive treatment group ($P<0.04$). Among the patients with ARF requiring RRT, mortality fell from 8.2% in the conventional group to 4.8% in the intensive treatment group ($P<0.007$). As patients in this study had a relatively low severity of illness (mean Acute Physiology and Chronic Health Evaluation [APACHE] II score of 9 in both groups), it is unknown whether this result is generalizable to patients with more severe illness. Nevertheless, despite this limitation, management of hyperglycemia is another important component of optimized medical care for critically ill patients.

Practical application

The preferred method for delivering nutrition is enteral feeding (see **Table 2**). Bowel rest in critically ill patients is accompanied by atrophy of the intestinal mucosa, which may compromise the immune function of this organ and increase the risk of bacterial translocation across the bowel wall. Enteral feedings are believed to reduce these complications, and formulas geared towards renal patients are generally recommended. These formulas contain a high, balanced protein content; are caloric-dense to limit volume; and limit potassium intake – all of which are desirable in patients with ARF.

If a patient is unable to tolerate enteral feeding, or enteral feeding is contraindicated (such as in bowel obstruction), then parenteral feeding should be initiated as early as possible. **Figure 1** provides one framework for designing a total parenteral nutrition (TPN) solution. Several comments need to be made regarding the composition of the TPN. First, the osmolality of the solution is dependent upon the sodium and potassium content. For patients who are oliguric and/or on intermittent hemodialysis, the general recommendation is to remove potassium and reduce the sodium content by 50%–75% depending on clinical factors (eg, hypotension, respiratory status, hyper- or hyponatremia). Second, the choice of sodium and potassium salts

Figure 1. Total parenteral nutrition worksheet.

TPN: total parenteral nutrition.
[a]For the equivalent of normal saline, enter 1.0; for the equivalent of half-normal saline, enter 0.5; for an intermediate solution, enter a number between 0.5 and 1.0; [b]accounts for sodium associated with protein content.

	Calculate caloric needs		
1	Patient's weight (kg)	☐	
2	Calories needed	☐	(30–40 kcal/kg)
3	Protein needed	☐	(1.5–2.0 g/kg)
4	Total calories (multiply lines 1 and 2)	☐	
5	Protein calories (multiply lines 1 and 3 then multiply by 4)	☐	
6	Non-protein calories (subtract line 5 from line 4)	☐	
7	Carbohydrate calories (multiply line 6 by 0.7)	☐	
8	Lipid calories (multiply line 6 by 0.3)	☐	
	Calculate caloric needs		
9	If stock solution concentrations are unknown, go to step 18		
10	Protein concentration	☐	(eg, 10 kcal/mL)
11	Carbohydrate concentration	☐	(eg, 2.38 kcal/mL)
12	Lipid concentration	☐	(eg, 2 kcal/mL)
13	Protein volume (divide line 5 by line 10)	☐	
14	Carbohydrate volume (divide line 7 by line 11)	☐	
15	Lipid volume (divide line 8 by line 12)	☐	
16	Desired additional volume	☐	
17	Total volume (add lines 13, 14, 15, and 16)	☐	
18	Assume total volume is 2,000 mL	☐	
	Calculate osmolality		
19	Total volume of TPN (from line 17 or 18)	☐	
20	Desired potassium content	☐	(0–40 mEq)
21	Desired osmolality[a]	☐	(0.5–1.0)
22	Sodium concentration[b] (multiply line 21 by 0.14)	☐	
23	Sodium content (multiply lines 19 and 22)	☐	
24	Net sodium content (subtract line 20 from line 23)	☐	

should take account of the clinical context of the patient. Typically, in patients with ARF the chloride salt is chosen as opposed to the phosphate or bicarbonate. Third, on TPN order forms there is an option to "balance" the solution using chloride or bicarbonate to maintain electrical neutrality. For the typical patient, chloride is the recommended choice unless there is a metabolic acidosis that needs to be compensated for. Fourth, the worksheet does not include other typical electrolytes, such as calcium and magnesium. The amount of these electrolytes depends on the individual patient; it is recommended to avoid all electrolytes except sodium chloride in patients on CRRT. Finally, multivitamins should be added to all TPN formulations.

References

1. Borum ML, Lynn J, Zhong Z et al. The effect of nutritional supplementation on survival in seriously ill hospitalized adults: an evaluation of the SUPPORT data. Study to Understand Prognoses and Preferences for Outcomes and Risks of Treatments. *J Am Geriatr Soc* 2000;48(5 Suppl.):S33–8.

2. Kierdorf HP. The nutritional management of acute renal failure in the intensive care unit. *New Horiz* 1995;3:699–707.

3. Clark WR, Mueller BA, Alaka KJ et al. A comparison of metabolic control by continuous and intermittent therapies in acute renal failure. *J Am Soc Nephrol* 1994;4:1413–20.

4. Maxvold NJ, Smoyer WE, Custer JR et al. Amino acid loss and nitrogen balance in critically ill children with acute renal failure: a prospective comparison between classic hemofiltration and hemofiltration with dialysis. *Crit Care Med* 2000;28:1161–5.

5. van den Berghe G, Wouters P, Weekers F et al. Intensive insulin therapy in the critically ill patients. *N Engl J Med* 2001;345:1359–67.

Part 7: Transplant patients

Edward Sha

A nephrologist should be consulted for all renal transplant patients admitted to the intensive care unit because these patients exhibit several distinct differences from other critically ill patients.

Acute renal failure

Renal transplant patients lack the typical physiologic renal reserves of other critically ill patients; therefore, they exhibit an increased risk for developing acute renal failure (ARF) similar to that of patients with chronic kidney disease. Transplant patients are also likely to be on medications such as calcineurin inhibitors that increase their vulnerability to volume depletion. Hence, attention should be paid to optimizing volume and cardiac status as well as avoiding potentially nephrotoxic agents.

Opportunistic infections

Transplant patients are at increased risk for opportunistic infections – although patients with renal transplants have the lowest risk of infection of all solid-organ recipients. **Figure 1** illustrates the time course following transplantation over which certain opportunistic infections may occur. It should be noted, however, that these data were originally published in 1981 and may not be representative of modern day transplantation using new immunosuppressive agents and prophylaxis regimens [1,2]. In the initial and early post-transplant period (<6 months), these patients are at increased risk of opportunistic viral infections such as cytomegalovirus, herpes simplex, and hepatitis B and C, because they have the potential to reactivate and present with a variety of clinical manifestations (see **Table 1**).

Table 1. Presentation and diagnostic tests for cytomegalovirus (CMV) and herpes simplex virus (HSV) infections.

GI: gastrointestinal; PCR: polymerase chain reaction.

Virus	Presentation	Diagnostic test
CMV	Pneumonitis Hepatitis GI tract involvement Glomerulopathy Leukopenia Arthritis	Rapid shell-viral culture CMV antigen CMV PCR
HSV	Pneumonitis Hepatitis GI tract involvement Encephalitis Skin involvement	Tzanck smear of lesions Viral culture HSV DNA PCR

Figure 1. Timeline of opportunistic infections in renal transplant patients.

CMV: cytomegalovirus; EBV: Epstein–Barr virus; HSV: herpes simplex virus; PTLD: post-transplant lymphoproliferative disease; RSV: respiratory syncytial virus; VSV: vesicular stomatitis virus. Reproduced with permission from Fishman, JA, Rubin RH. Infection in organ-transplant recipients. *N Engl J Med* 1998;338:1741–51. Copyright © 2004 Massachusetts Medical Society. All rights reserved.

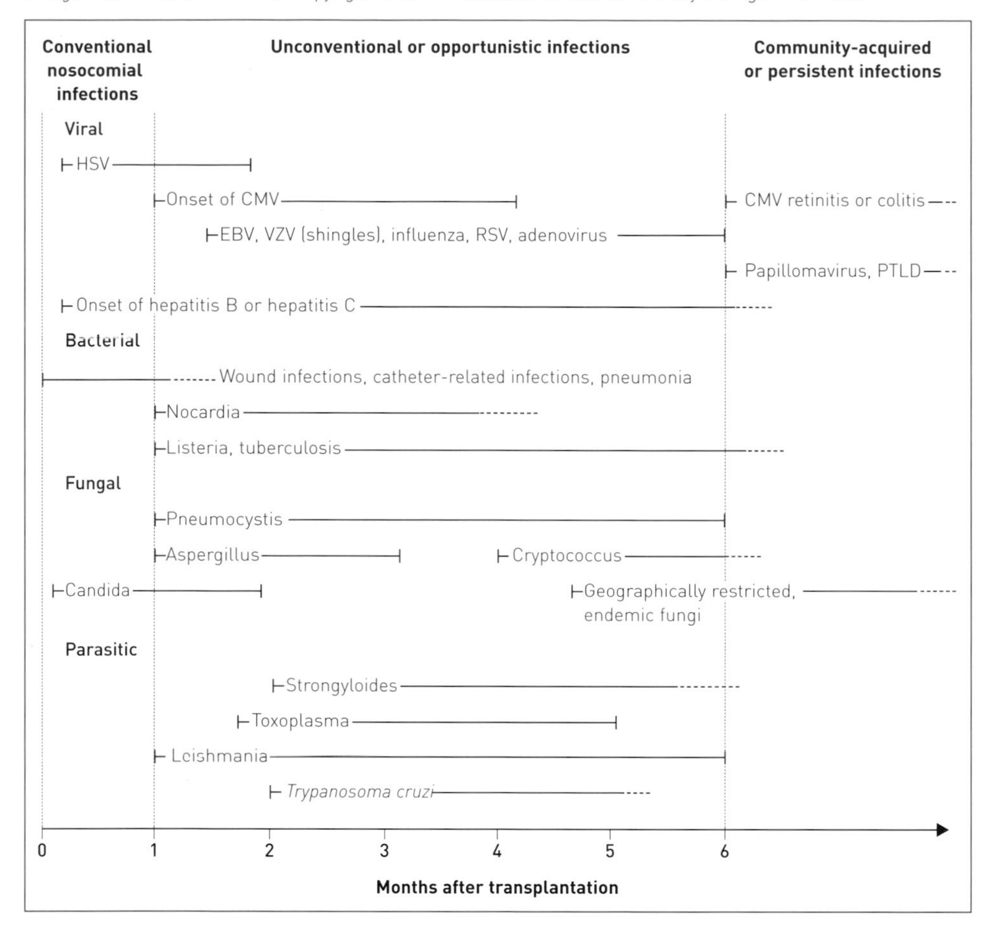

In patients with anti-hepatitis C virus antibodies prior to renal transplantation, 20%–60% will develop liver disease, although this does not have a significant impact on renal graft or patient survival. Fungal infections occur in up to 10% of renal transplant patients, with *Candida albicans* being the most common, causatory organism. Portals of entry typically involve the gastrointestinal or urinary tracts, and intravascular catheters. *Pneumocystis carinii* should be suspected when respiratory symptoms are out of proportion to findings on physical examination and when patients are not receiving prophylaxis or have ongoing rejection issues. In the late post-transplant period (>6 months), patients develop infections typical of the general population.

Immunosuppressive agents

The issue of continuing infected patients on immunosuppressive agents should be decided on a case-by-case basis as there are few published data. Most treating physicians would discontinue OKT3, mycophenolate mofetil, and azathioprine. Because calcineurin inhibitors, such as cyclosporine and tacrolimus, have a vasoconstrictive effect, reducing the dose of these medications is prudent in transplant patients admitted to the intensive care unit. If the decision is made to continue with these or other agents, their levels should be monitored carefully to ensure that they remain in the therapeutic range. Steroids are typically continued due to the risk of precipitating an Addisonian crisis. It is strongly recommended that a nephrologist experienced in caring for transplant patients be consulted.

References

1. Fishman JA, Rubin RH. Infection in organ-transplant recipients. *N Engl J Med* 1998;338:1741–51.
2. Rubin RH, Wolfson JS, Cosimi AB et al. Infection in the renal transplant recipient. *Am J Med* 1981;70:405–11.

Section 3

Acute renal failure

Part 1: Approach to acute renal failure

Bruce A Molitoris

Introduction

Acute renal failure (ARF) is defined as a decline in glomerular filtration rate (GFR) sufficient to cause retention of nitrogenous wastes (creatinine and blood urea nitrogen [BUN]). Unfortunately, there is no standard definition of the magnitude of rise in creatinine or BUN that constitutes a diagnosis of ARF. This lack of rigid standard nomenclature for characterization of ARF results from the heterogeneous patient population with regards to severity of injury, clinical presentation, comorbid disease processes, incidence, and etiologies of ARF. One useful way to classify ARF is as mild, moderate, or severe (see **Figure 1**), since the severity of ARF increases with decreasing GFR. More severe ARF is associated with the need for renal replacement therapy and with an increased mortality rate [1,2]. However, at present, little attention is paid to quantifying the extent of injury in ARF. This is in large part due to the lack of availability of appropriate and easy-to-use techniques and parameters, a situation that contrasts markedly with that for myocardial ischemic injury (**Table 1**).

Oliguria and anuria are also frequent and important indicators of renal dysfunction, especially in the acute setting [3]. In adults, oliguria is defined as a urine output of <400 mL/day or <20 mL/h. In children, oliguria is defined as a urine output of <0.8 mL/kg/h. Anuria refers to the total cessation of urine output. Although both oliguria and anuria require rapid medical attention, anuria is at the most severe end of the spectrum

Figure 1. Spectrum of acute renal failure.
GFR: glomerular filtration rate; RRT: renal replacement therapy; S_{CR}: serum creatinine.

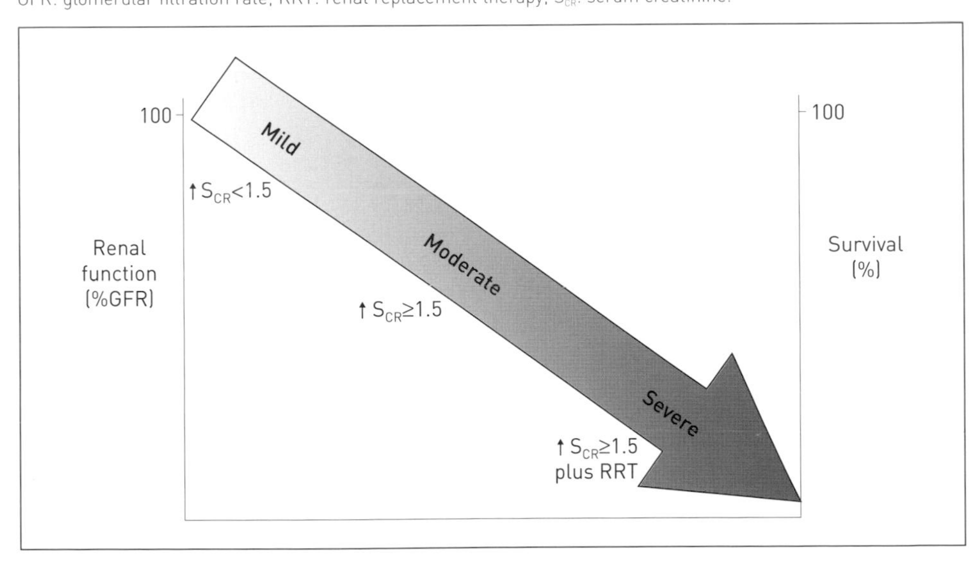

Table 1. Contrasting myocardial infarction and ischemic acute renal failure (ARF).

ECG: electrocardiogram; ER: emergency room; FENa: fractional excretion of sodium; UA: urinalysis.

Characteristic	Myocardial infarction	Ischemic ARF
Precursor	Angina	Prerenal azotemia
Detection - Early - Late	 ECG, enzymes Echo	 UA, FENa ↑ Serum creatinine
Diagnosis	ER	1–2 days
Therapy	Effective	Supportive
Effect of toxins	+/–	+++

Table 2. Etiology of anuria.

Bilateral renal artery occlusion
Bilateral renal vein occlusion
Complete obstruction of both ureters
Complete obstruction of the urethra
Cortical necrosis secondary to severe ischemia (rare)
Rapidly progressive glomerulonephritis (rare)

and constitutes a true medical emergency. Anuria occurs when the GFR is zero as a result of either complete occlusion of arterial or venous blood flow, or complete obstruction of urine flow (**Table 2**). ARF is usually subclassified into anuric, oliguric, and nonoliguric subtypes, as patients with nonoliguric ARF usually have a better prognosis. This may well relate to a less severe insult or a higher incidence of nephrotoxin-induced ARF in the nonoliguric group.

The overall incidence of ARF in the hospital setting is 3%–5%, but there are marked differences within different departments, reflecting variations in the underlying disease process (**Figure 2**). ARF in the intensive care unit (ICU) is common (~13% of all admissions to the ICU present with ARF), often multifactorial, and associated with a poor prognosis [4]. Mortality rates in ARF vary from <10% in patients with prerenal azotemia to approximately 80% in patients with ARF and multiple organ dysfunction syndrome. Several studies have now demonstrated that the presence of ARF is an independent predictor of a markedly increased mortality rate irrespective of the underlying physiologic status (Acute Physiology and Chronic Health Evaluation [APACHE] II score) of the patient. Therefore, prevention and the early diagnosis/treatment of ARF are of paramount importance in ICU patients [5,6]. Indeed, the presence of ARF should elicit as urgent a response as myocardial ischemia.

Etiology of acute renal failure

The etiologies, functional localizations, and histologic classifications of ARF are shown in **Figure 3**, together with specific examples. The etiology of ARF in the ICU patient is different from that in the ward patient, with a higher incidence of acute tubular necrosis (ATN) and less prerenal azotemia. (ARF resulting from hypoperfusion or nephrotoxins has been termed ATN by pathologists, based on the occasional occurrence of mild patchy sites of necrosis

Figure 2. Frequency of acute renal failure in selected hospital settings.

CABG: coronary artery bypass graft; ICU: intensive care unit.

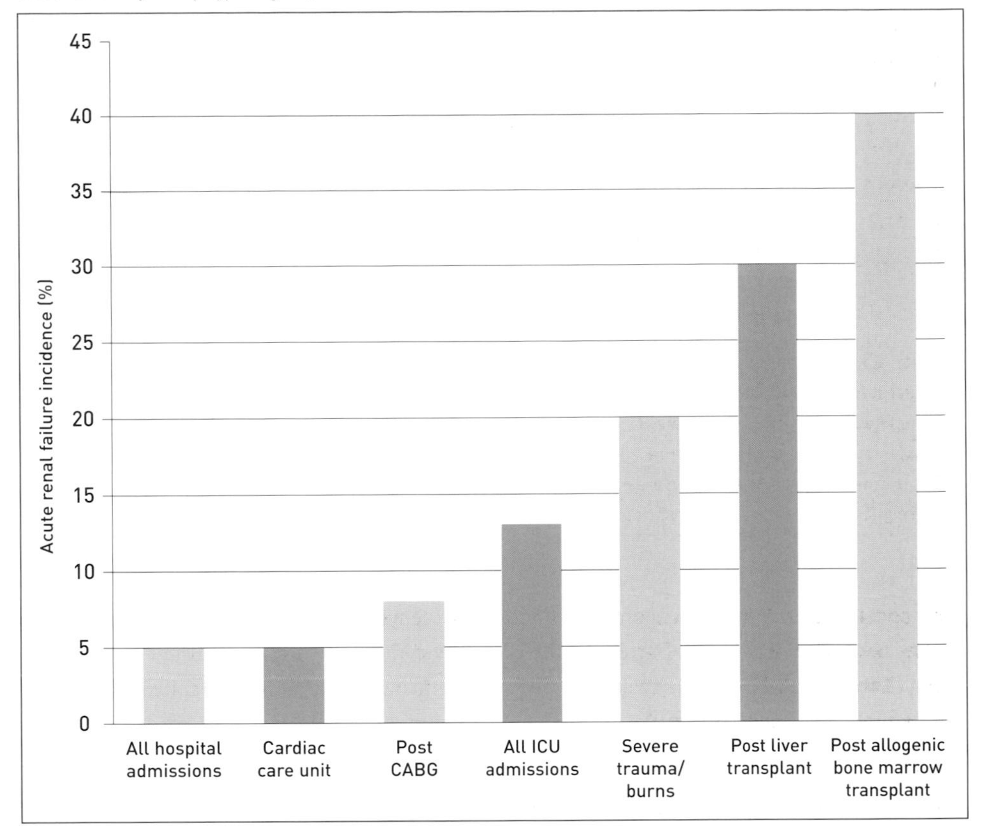

on pathologic evaluation.) Furthermore, the severity and mortality of ARF in ICU patients are markedly higher than in patients acquiring ARF in the ward or as outpatients.

Diagnosis of ARF is functionally divided into prerenal, intrarenal, and postrenal etiologies.

Prerenal etiologies of acute renal failure

Prerenal etiologies present as diminished blood flow to the kidney, resulting in diminished GFR. Generally, they occur in the absence of any overt renal pathology.

Prerenal azotemia

Prerenal azotemia is a common etiology of ARF, and a large percentage of patients with ATN initially experience a phase of prerenal azotemia [7]. Prerenal azotemia is rapidly reversible if the underlying cause can be corrected before cellular injury has occurred, and consequently it is associated with low morbidity and mortality (<10%), assuming prompt diagnosis and treatment. Prerenal azotemia results from mild to moderate reductions in renal blood flow, primarily due to a reduction in the effective arterial volume (EAV) (**Table 3**). EAV is defined

Figure 3. Etiology of acute renal failure in intensive care unit patients.
NSAID: nonsteroidal anti-inflammatory drug.

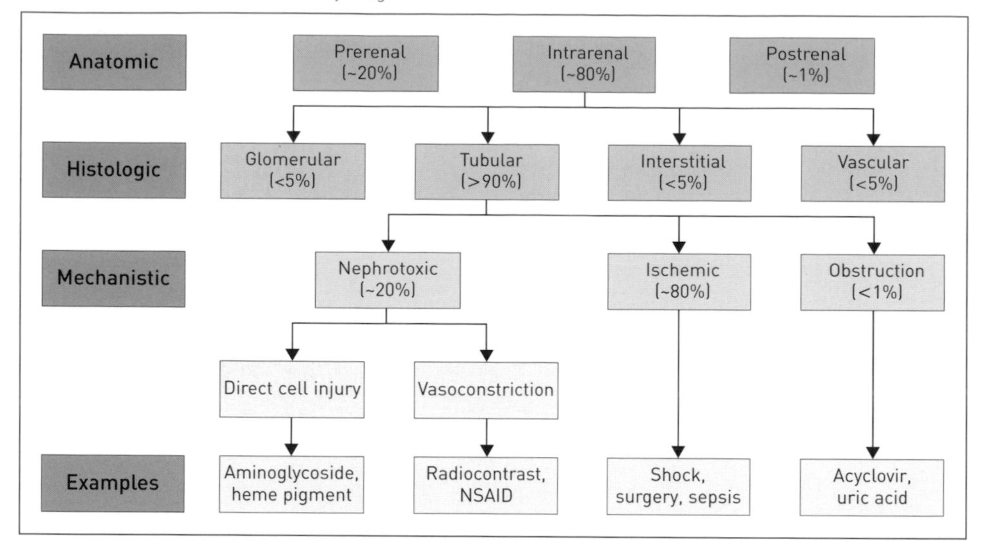

as the amount of arterial blood effectively perfusing vital organs. The determinants of EAV include cardiac output and vascular resistance. Although venous and interstitial volumes can be estimated by careful physical examination, EAV cannot. Furthermore, the EAV can be reduced when total body volume status is reduced, normal, or increased (**Table 3**). For example, hemorrhage results in a reduced arterial volume and reduced cardiac output in a state of high vascular resistance. On the other hand, in congestive heart failure the reduced cardiac output is directly responsible (see **Table 1** in **Section 2, Part 2**, *page 62*). Hence, surrogate measures, including invasive pulmonary atrial monitoring and determination of the fractional excretion (FE) of sodium (FENa), are required to estimate effective arterial volume. An FENa <1% is generally considered indicative of prerenal azotemia as the etiology of ARF (**Table 4**). As a result of reduced EAV, urine flow decreases and there is increased proximal tubule affinity for sodium secondary to increased angiotensin II and adrenergic-mediated vasoconstriction. Simultaneously, enhanced aldosterone production leads to increased distal sodium reabsorption. The end result is a low FENa as long as the tubular epithelium remains intact and fully functional.

However, there are circumstances in which a paradoxically high FENa is obtained despite the presence of prerenal azotemia. Exceptions to this rule do occur in patients who have a high FENa in the absence of cellular injury. For example, patients who have received diuretics within the previous 24 hours, those who have recently received mannitol, those with chronic kidney disease with a high baseline urinary sodium excretion, those with glucosuria, and those presenting with alkaline urine.

Conversely, a low FENa does not always indicate prerenal azotemia. A low FENa is also obtained in the early stages of obstruction, acute glomerular nephritis, pigment nephropathy, and intrinsic ARF induced by radiographic contrast agents.

Table 3. Reduced effective arterial volume, as a cause of prerenal azotemia, occurs in states of reduced, normal, or increased total body volume.

Body fluid status reduced	Body fluid status normal	Body fluid status increased
Hemorrhage	Sepsis	Congestive heart failure
Burns	Cirrhosis	Aortic stenosis
Surgery	Anaphylaxis	Reduced serum albumin
Dehydration	Vasodilatory drugs	Cor pulmonale
Diuretics	Anesthetic agents	Ascites
Gastrointestinal losses		Venocaval syndromes

Table 4. Urinary diagnostic indices in acute renal failure.

ATN: acute tubular necrosis; FE: fractional excretion.

Test	Prerenal	ATN
Urinalysis	Hyaline casts	Abnormal
Specific gravity	>1.020	~1.010
Urinary osmolality (mOsm/kg H_2O)	>500	~300
Urinary Na^+ (mEq/L)	<20	>40
FENa (%)	<1	>2
FE uric acid (%)	<7	>15
FE lithium (%)	<7	>20
FE urea (%)	<35	>50

A reduced effective arterial volume state also stimulates antidiuretic hormone (ADH) release. ADH results in increased distal water and urea nitrogen (UN) reabsorption. Some investigators have used a low FE of UN (FEUN) as a diagnostic indicator of prerenal azotemia [8]. Measuring FEUN is of particular use in patients having received a diuretic within 24 hours or in states of high-urinary-output prerenal azotemia, as occur in cases of high solute clearance by the kidney. For example, burn and trauma patients can be prerenal yet have urine outputs in the 1–2 L range. Other useful indicators of prerenal azotemia include the FE of lithium and the BUN to creatinine ratio, which increases as filtered urinary BUN is reabsorbed distally and therefore retained while filtered creatinine is excreted. Lithium is primarily reabsorbed by the proximal tubule, and therefore lithium reabsorption can be used to selectively evaluate proximal tubule function. Other useful indicators of prerenal azotemia are listed in **Table 4**. In patients with metabolic alkalosis, the FE of chloride ions should be used.

Diagnosing prerenal azotemia in the chronic kidney disease patient with a high baseline sodium excretion is probably the most significant challenge for clinicians. Since rapid adaptation to a reduced EAV is not possible in such patients, the FENa remains high and the clinician will often erroneously diagnose ATN. These patients require urgent correction of their volume status, and respond to hydration with an increase in GFR and a decrease in serum creatinine. Finally, if the patient has had diuretics within the previous 24 hours it is still worthwhile measuring the FENa since a low value is very helpful as evidence of prerenal azotemia.

Table 5. Urinalysis in acute renal failure.

AIN: acute interstitial nephritis; ATN: acute tubular necrosis; GN: glomerulonephritis; RBC: red blood cell; WBC: white blood cell.

	Protein	WBC casts	RBC casts	Urinary Na^+	Miscellaneous
Prerenal	–	–	–	↓	Granular casts
ATN	–	–	–	↑	Muddy brown casts
GN nephrotic	+++	+/–	+/–	↓	
GN nephritic	++	++	++	↓	
AIN	+	+/–	+/–	↑	Eosinophils in urine
Pyelonephritis	+	++	+/–	↑	
Obstruction	–	–	–	↓ early ↑ late	Crystals

Intrarenal causes of acute renal failure

A wide spectrum of renal disease processes can cause intrarenal ARF (**Figure 3**). Ischemia and nephrotoxins are responsible for the majority of cases in the ICU, but consideration must be given to all potential etiologies [9]. Urinalysis is extremely important in determining the cause of ARF (**Table 5**) [10]. A high urine protein (albumin, as measured by dipstick) is indicative of a glomerular problem, but is also observed in patients with fever or severe elevations in blood pressure. Urinary white blood cells and casts are seen in several disease processes that can cause ARF, and urinary eosinophils are suggestive of either acute interstitial nephritis (AIN) or atheroembolic disease. Fever and rash with an elevated peripheral eosinophil count, in conjunction with urinary eosinophils, are highly suggestive of AIN, but are seen in less than half of cases. Dysmorphic red blood cells and casts are seen in a wide range of disease processes, but are suggestive of nephritic (inflammatory) glomerular processes and vasculitides.

Prerenal azotemia and ischemic ARF represent two ends of a spectrum of reduced renal perfusion in which the extent and duration of decreases in renal blood flow (RBF) determine the pathologic outcome. Hence, it is essential to rapidly diagnose and treat prerenal azotemia before it progresses, as the clinical outcome of ischemic ATN remains poor. The tubular cell dysfunction characteristic of ATN is responsible for the high FENa, limited ability to excrete protons, and reduced renal concentrating ability seen in ischemic ARF. Recovery of tubular function is possible, given early administration of fluids, as tubular cells are able to undergo repair and differentiation, proliferation, and repopulation from stem cells, resulting in improved GFR.

Nephrotoxin-induced tubular cell injury

Nephrotoxins induce tubular cell injury by several primary mechanisms (**Figure 3**):

- direct tubular cell injury (eg, aminoglycosides, amphotericin, heavy metals, foscarnet, pentamidine, and cisplatin)
- indirect tubular cell injury via vasoconstriction and subsequent reductions in RBF (eg, nonsteroidal anti-inflammatory drugs [NSAIDs])

- crystal-induced tubular obstruction (eg, uric acid, acyclovir, sulfonamides, methotrexate, triamterene, and ethylene glycol)

Many nephrotoxins (eg, radiographic contrast agents, cyclosporin A, and heme pigments) cause both direct cellular toxicity and vasoconstriction. In addition, efferent vasodilation by angiotensin II receptor antagonists or angiotensin-converting enzyme inhibitors can lead to a reduced GFR secondary to a reduced filtration fraction with near normal RBF. This is characteristically rapidly reversible if detected early and the offending agent withdrawn. Furthermore, certain agents (eg, gold, penicillamine, and some NSAIDs) induce specific glomerulopathies. Finally, any drug can induce interstitial nephritis by an idiosyncratic immune-mediated mechanism, with methicillin being the classic example.

Synergistic interactions between nephrotoxins and prerenal azotemia

Although there is a natural tendency to look for one specific cause, it is often the case that two or more factors combine in a synergistic fashion to induce oliguria and renal injury. ARF in such patients is termed "multifactorial ARF". This is especially common in ICU patients due to their multifactorial disease processes and need for multiple tests and therapies [11]. Examples include interactions between nephrotoxins (including aminoglycosides, radiographic contrast agents, cyclosporin A, cisplatin, uric acid, and heme pigments) and reduced EAV or ischemia (**Figure 4**). In the case of aminoglycosides, renal hypoperfusion increases the incidence of ARF from approximately 5% to 30%–50% (**Figure 5**). Therefore, it is essential to ensure adequate renal perfusion by correcting any deficit in volume status and maximizing RBF prior to administering potential nephrotoxins. This is also true in the prevention of ARF from endogenous nephrotoxic compounds such as heme pigments and uric acid.

Although the incidence of glomerulonephritis (GN), AIN, pyelonephritis, vasculitis, and extrarenal obstruction in the ICU patient is low, it is important to aggressively evaluate the patient for these treatable causes of ARF. AIN, in particular, should be suspected in a patient with ARF occurring during a course of antibiotics. The triad of fever, a new rash, and an increased peripheral eosinophil count, especially with pyuria and eosinophils in the urine, is diagnostic of AIN.

Anuria and acute renal failure

Anuria is the absolute lack of urine production [3]. The diagnosis requires placement of a urinary catheter to drain previously formed urine, and to document the lack of new urine production. Although there are several potential causes, the primary cause is total urinary obstruction. This could occur at the level of the ureters, as with retroperitoneal fibrosis, or at the level of the urethra. Total occlusion of the renal arteries or renal venous system bilaterally by thrombosis or an embolism can also result in total lack of urine flow. Finally, severe forms of hypoperfusion resulting in cortical necrosis or severe rapidly progressive GN can also produce this syndrome. Whatever the cause, the diagnostic and therapeutic approach must be fast and efficient. Since occlusion of either the urinary tract or the renal vascular system is potentially reversible, each may need to be ruled out.

Figure 4. Synergistic interaction between ischemia and nephrotoxins.
Reproduced with permission from Molitoris BA. Cell biology of aminoglycoside nephrotoxicity: newer aspects. *Curr Opin Nephrol Hypertens* 1997;6:384–8.

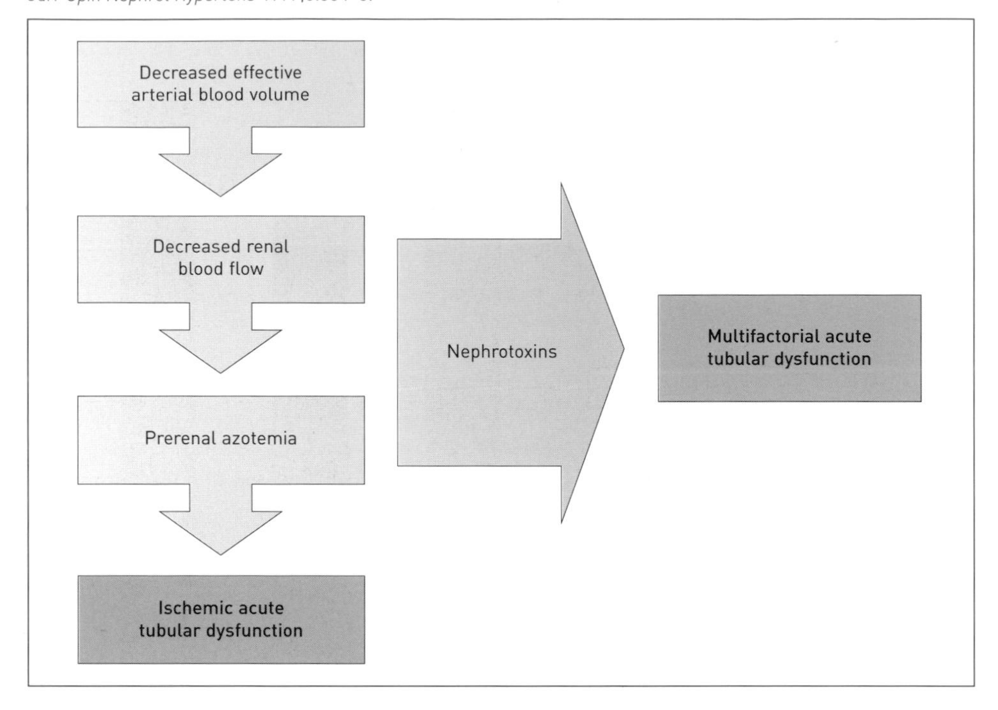

Approach to the patient with acute renal failure

As ARF can result from a wide range of clinical insults, the approach involves a meticulous history, complete physical examination, and the efficient and cost-effective utilization of the laboratory to establish the diagnosis and to direct therapy [12]. It is of paramount importance to rapidly differentiate prerenal azotemia from ischemic ARF, as failure to do this can result in the development of established ARF in patients presenting with prerenal azotemia. It is of particular importance during the history and physical examination to pay close attention to the volume status of the patient and any recent exposure to potential nephrotoxins. Reviewing the patient's hospital pharmacological records and anesthesia notes is essential.

In all patients, a careful urinalysis (UA) should be conducted, as this will yield critical diagnostic information, especially in intrarenal causes of ARF. For example, in ischemia- or nephrotoxin-induced ARF, the UA shows mild proteinuria and pigmented granular casts. However, in acute GN there is a high protein content, white blood cells, erythrocytes, and cellular casts. In interstitial nephritis there is mild to moderate proteinuria, leukocytes, erythrocytes, and eosinophils. The presence of heme positivity on the dipstick and no erythrocytes in the urine suggests the presence of myoglobin or hemoglobin, indicating either rhabdomyolysis or hemolysis. The presence of eosinophils is suggestive of acute interstitial nephritis, but can also be seen in renal atheroembolism or pyelonephritis. Specific urinary crystals can also be indicative of causes of ARF. For example, oxalate crystals are seen in

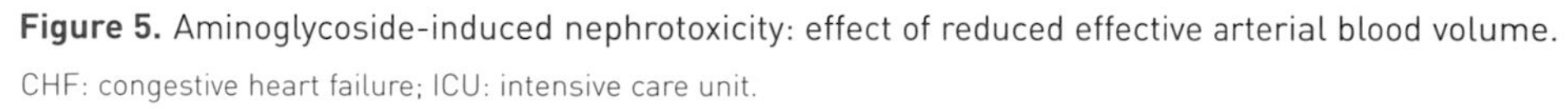
Figure 5. Aminoglycoside-induced nephrotoxicity: effect of reduced effective arterial blood volume.
CHF: congestive heart failure; ICU: intensive care unit.

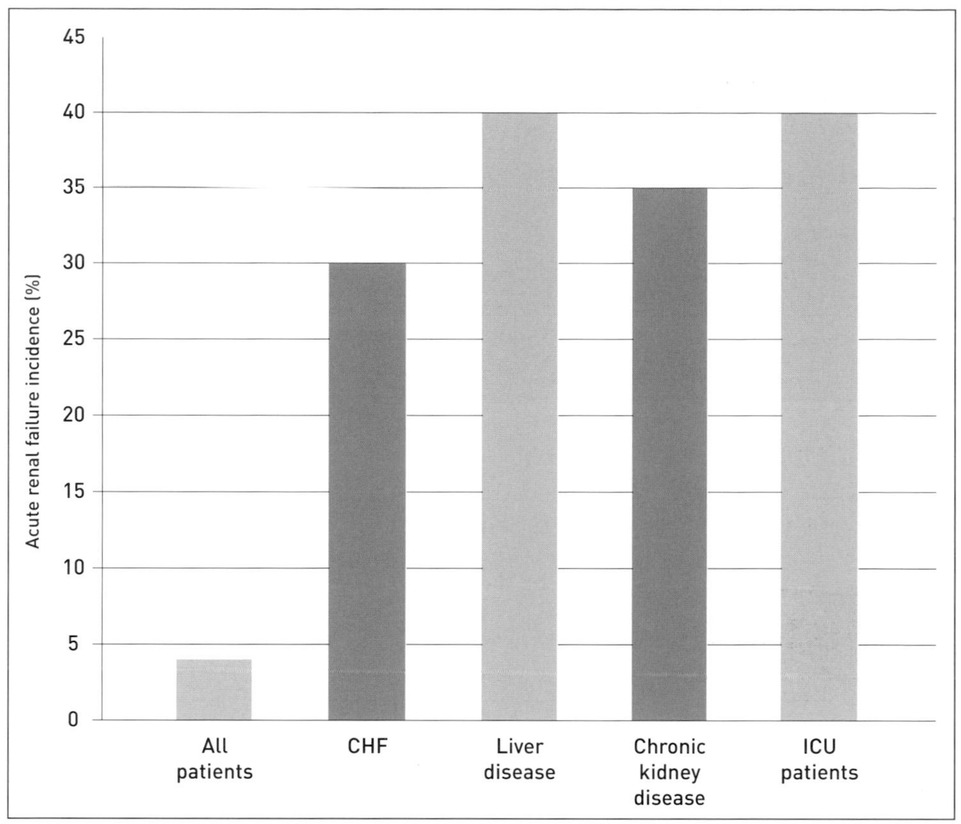

cases of ethylene glycol ingestion, and uric acid crystals are seem in cases of tumor lysis syndrome. Urinary diagnostic indices should be sent to the laboratory in any case where prerenal azotemia is in the differential diagnosis. Very high serum creatinine (eg, 13 mg/dL) does not preclude the diagnosis of prerenal azotemia.

Renal ultrasound should be carried out in most cases of ARF. Ultrasound is the preferred imaging modality for identifying obstruction, as use of radiocontrast agents could be potentially harmful and cause the clinical situation to deteriorate. Besides evaluating for obstruction, the ultrasound can give valuable information regarding kidney size, and the size, quality, and quantity of renal parenchyma. Thinning of the renal cortex or increased echogenicity is consistent with reduced function and chronicity of the disease process. If the clinical situation dictates evaluation of the renal vasculature then isotopic scans, Doppler flow studies, or angiography should be utilized depending upon the clinical situation and urgency of diagnosis. In general, angiography should be avoided because of the potential for contrast-induced nephrotoxicity. However, there are instances when angiography is essential, such as in cases of renal artery thrombosis.

Table 6. Minimizing the risk of development of acute renal failure.

Identification of high-risk patients
Use of volume expansion
Preoperative optimization of cardiovascular hemodynamics in selected high-risk patients
Aggressive surveillance of renal function in high-risk patients
Minimizing use of nephrotoxins
Changing dosage schedule
Modifying formulation of nephrotoxins
Minimizing use and length of invasive lines and in-dwelling catheters to avoid nosocomial infection

Prevention, management, and nondialytic treatment of acute renal failure

Overall, despite improvements in dialysis and intensive care, the average mortality rate in patients with ARF has declined very little since the advent of dialysis. Although during this time there have been great advances in our understanding of the pathophysiology of ARF, and especially ischemic ARF, our ability to translate this knowledge into clinical benefit has been limited, for a number of reasons. These include the lack of early diagnosis and treatment, underpowered clinical studies, using an agent with a single therapeutic target, and lack of adequate dialysis in the study population.

Prevention of ARF is of paramount importance (**Table 6**), and a number of risk factors have been identified, including volume depletion or hypoperfusion, preexisting renal disease, and exposure to vasoconstricting drugs such as NSAIDs (**Table 7**). Avoiding these agents or situations is essential. It is also important to limit the use of nephrotoxins such as aminoglycosides, and to use alternative medications when possible, especially in high-risk patients. Furthermore, since many cases of ischemic or nephrotoxic ARF result from sepsis or use of a nephrotoxic antibiotic, respectively, limiting infections is an important preventive strategy.

Treatment of established ARF has centered on the use of loop diuretics or dopamine. Both loop diuretics and dopamine have been used alone or in combination to convert oliguric to nonoliguric ARF. Conversion can be clinically important, as increasing urine output can minimize the occurrence of volume overload and hyperkalemia. This in turn may reduce the need for early dialysis and allow for adequate nutritional support. Both agents, either alone or in combination, should be started as soon as oliguria is diagnosed, as it is generally felt – but not proven – that the response rate is higher the earlier they are started. While both loop diuretics and low-dose dopamine (<3 μg/kg body weight/min) are known to increase urine output, neither increases GFR and neither has been shown to enhance recovery rates or clinical outcomes. The approach to using diuretics in ARF is outlined in **Section 2, Part 3**.

To date the only beneficial therapy for ATN has been increased dialytic support [1]. This is reviewed in **Section 4, Part 1**.

Table 7. Risk factors for acute renal failure.

Reduced effective arterial volume:
- Volume depletion
- Congestive heart failure
- Liver disease
- Nephrotic syndrome
- Chronic kidney disease
Existing renal dysfunction
Nonsteroidal anti-inflammatory drugs
Advanced age
Diabetes mellitus

References

1. Schiffl H, Lang SM, Fischer R. Daily hemodialysis and the outcome of acute renal failure. *N Engl J Med* 2002;346:305–10.
2. Mehta RL, Pascual MT, Gruta CG et al. Refining predictive models in critically ill patients with acute renal failure. *J Am Soc Nephrol* 2002;13:1350–7.
3. Klahr S, Miller SB. Acute oliguria. *N Engl J Med* 1998;338:671–5.
4. Thadhani R, Pascual M, Bonventre JV. Acute renal failure. *N Engl J Med* 1996;334:1448–60.
5. Murray PT, Le Gall JR, Dos Reis Miranda D et al. Physiologic endpoints (efficacy) for acute renal failure studies. *Curr Opin Crit Care* 2002;8:519–25.
6. Sutton TA, Molitoris BA. Mechanisms of cellular injury in ischemic acute renal failure. *Semin Nephrol* 1998;18:490–7.
7. Blantz RC. Pathophysiology of pre-renal azotemia. *Kidney Int* 1998;53:512–23.
8. Carvounis CP, Nisar S, Guro-Razuman S. Significance of the fractional excretion of urea in the differential diagnosis of acute renal failure. *Kidney Int* 2002;62:2223–9.
9. Liano F, Pascual J. Epidemiology of acute renal failure: a prospective, multicenter, community-based study. Madrid Acute Renal Failure Study Group. *Kidney Int* 1996;50:811–8.
10. Miller TR, Anderson RJ, Linas SL et al. Urinary diagnostic indices in acute renal failure: a prospective study. *Ann Intern Med* 1978;89:47–50.
11. Molitoris BA. Cell biology of aminoglycoside nephrotoxicity: newer aspects. *Curr Opin Nephrol Hypertens* 1997;6:384–8.
12. Nolan CR, Anderson RJ. Hospital-acquired acute renal failure. *J Am Soc Nephrol* 1998;9:710–8.

Part 2: Outcomes and prognosis

Edward Sha

Introduction

The overall outcome of critically ill patients with acute renal failure (ARF) remains poor, with mortality rates ranging between 40% and 90% depending on the patient population being studied. However, with improvements in the management of critically ill patients and in renal replacement therapies, the overall survival rate has increased; however, this improvement has been partially obscured by changes in the patient population. Here in **Part 2** we will review the current outcomes of critically ill patients with ARF, the tools available to determine prognosis, and how well these prognostic tools perform.

Outcomes

As a population, critically ill patients have a high mortality rate, ranging between 10% and 20%. However, if they develop ARF, their mortality rate jumps more than fourfold. Even when matched for disease severity and demographic factors, patients with ARF continue to have an almost twofold higher mortality rate, and this difference suggests that ARF is an independent risk factor for morbidity and mortality. Among patients with ARF, the need for renal replacement therapy increases the mortality rate an additional 1.5-fold compared with patients who have ARF alone.

ARF in the intensive care unit (ICU) rarely presents as an isolated disease process; it typically presents as part of the multiple organ dysfunction syndrome (MODS). Various studies have demonstrated a significant association between mortality and the following concomitant medical conditions: respiratory failure, circulatory failure, hepatic dysfunction, altered neurologic status, and hematologic or coagulation abnormalities. Emphasizing this point is the observation that the number of failing organs (including kidneys) correlates with mortality rate (**Figure 1**).

The etiology of ARF in these critically ill patients was predominantly acute tubular necrosis (ATN), which is the most common etiology in the ICU. Interestingly, sepsis as a discrete entity has rarely been shown to be a significant risk factor for mortality, possibly because it typically presents as part of MODS.

For postoperative patients, the development of ARF is associated with mortality rates of 40%–100%, with the highest rate in those undergoing major cardiovascular or thoracic surgery. Chertow and colleagues [1] performed a prospective, cohort study of veterans undergoing coronary bypass or valvular heart surgery to determine preoperative risk factors for the development of ARF (defined as a 50% increase in serum creatinine). They found that this group of patients had a mortality rate of 63.7% compared with a mortality rate of 4.3% in

Figure 1. Mortality rate increases proportional to the number of dysfunctional organs.

SOFA: Sequential Organ Failure Assessment.

[a]Graph reproduced with permission from Ferreira FL, Bota DP, Bross A et al. Serial evaluation of the SOFA score to predict outcome in critically ill patients. *JAMA* 2001;286:1754–8. *Copyright ©2004, American Medical Association.* All rights reserved.

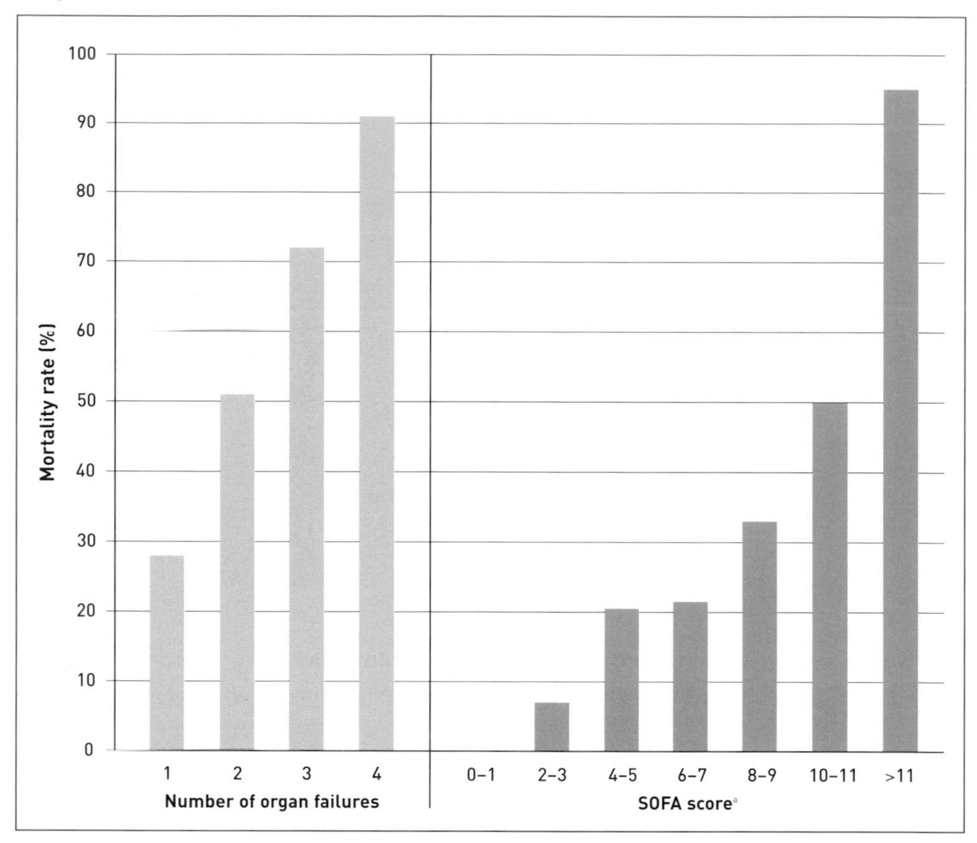

patients who did not develop ARF. In order to determine the preoperative risk for developing ARF requiring dialysis, they derived the classification algorithm depicted in **Figure 2**.

The presence of chronic kidney disease also adversely affects the outcome of critically ill patients. In a study by Chertow and colleagues [1], the risk of developing ARF, with its associated mortality risk, was inversely related to the patient's baseline renal function. It increased from 0.5% in patients with baseline creatinine <1 mg/dL to 4.9% in patients with baseline creatinine between 2.0 mg/dL and 2.9 mg/dL. Older age was also associated with the risk of developing ARF, which increased from 0% in patients aged <40 years undergoing coronary artery bypass to 1.8% in patients >80 years. Advanced age is a known surgical risk factor, but it is unclear why this correlation is not seen in a broader, nonsurgical, intensive care population with ARF. It is possible that these surgical patients represent a more homogenous population in which age is a greater risk factor for mortality.

Because it would be considered unethical to withhold dialysis, studies to assess whether renal replacement therapy itself contributes to increased mortality cannot be performed.

Figure 2. Preoperative risk stratification for acute renal failure.

CrCl: creatinine clearance; NYHA: New York Heart Association; PVD: peripheral vascular disease. Reproduced with permission from Chertow GM, Lazarus JM, Christiansen CL et al. Preoperative renal risk stratification. *Circulation* 1997;95:878–84.

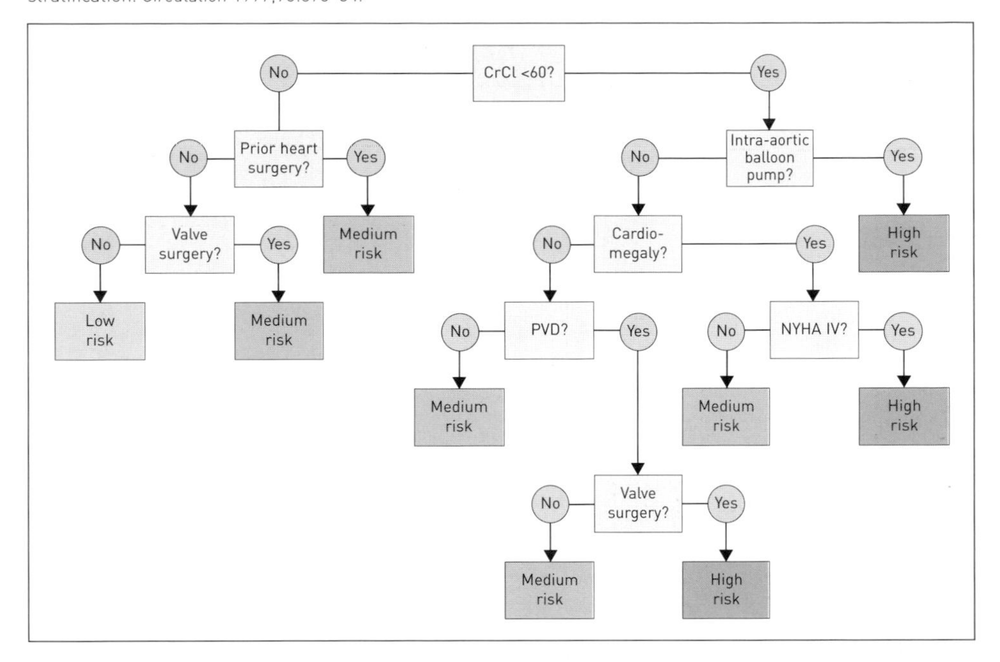

However, a strong argument can be made that mortality rates have improved since the development of dialysis, transforming severe ARF from a near-uniformly fatal condition into a manageable disease process. If that is indeed the case, then the pressing issue becomes whether there are aspects of dialysis that can be improved upon to reduce these patients' mortality risk. This topic is discussed in **Section 4, Part 1**.

Despite the availability of renal replacement therapies and improvements in medical practices within ICUs over the last several decades, the mortality rate of patients with ARF has remained high. Studies published in the 1980s suggested that no improvements had occurred in the mortality rate for critically ill patients with ARF up to that time period; some even suggested that it had worsened. However, more recent studies have shown a significant improvement in mortality. In a retrospective review of the Mayo Clinic experience [2], critically ill patients requiring dialysis were analyzed from two separate time periods 1977–1979 and 1991–1993. Patients from the latter time period were significantly older (mean 64.1 years vs. 58.6 years), were more likely to survive (52% vs. 32%), and had a higher severity of illness as determined by the Acute Physiology and Chronic Health Evaluation [APACHE] II score of nonsurvivors (29.4 vs. 28.2). In fact, several studies [2–4] have demonstrated that the age of critically-ill patients with ARF and the severity of illness have increased. In other words, the mortality rate for critically ill patients with ARF has improved; however, changes in the patient population have obscured this improvement in patient outcomes. When factors such as age and severity of disease are adjusted for, it becomes clear that the mortality rate has significantly improved.

Table 1. Long-term renal function depends on the underlying cause of acute renal failure.
HUS: hemolytic uremic syndrome; TTP: thrombotic thrombocytopenic purpura.

Renal function after 5 years	Etiology of acute renal failure
Good	Henoch–Schönlein purpura
↓	Allergic interstitial nephritis
	Endocapillary proliferative glomerulonephritis
	Acute tubular necrosis (ischemia, nephrotoxins, etc.)
	Diffuse lupus nephritis
	Membranoproliferative glomerulonephritis
	TTP/HUS
	Extracapillary proliferative glomerulonephritis
Bad	Acute cortical necrosis

The majority of patients in the ICU with ARF have a reasonably good outcome if they survive the hospitalization: their post-hospitalization mortality risk is similar to that of other critically ill patients. However, preservation of their renal function is dependent upon the underlying etiology of their ARF (**Table 1**).

The majority of patients with normal renal function prior to the insult who suffer tubular damage, such as ATN or allergic interstitial nephritis, have normal renal function 5 years later. However, nearly all patients who experience thrombotic microangiopathy or acute cortical necrosis continue to require chronic dialysis after 5 years. The 5-year outcome for patients with glomerular damage varies depending on the etiology, being worst in the case of extracapillary proliferative glomerulonephritis and best for Henoch–Schönlein purpura. In addition, ARF occurring in the setting of chronic kidney disease is more likely to result in worsening of the already reduced glomerular filtration rate and perhaps more rapid progression to end-stage renal disease.

Prognostic tools

Outcome and prognosis are related concepts. Outcome refers to the end result of a disease process or procedure, and it is often used to assess the effectiveness of a particular treatment. Prognosis is the ability to discern the outcome based on the available evidence. Prognostic information is important to patients and their families to help them make informed decisions and to prepare them for likely outcomes. Similarly, prognostic information is important to physicians and the medical system in order to guide treatment decisions, maximize the patient's chances of an optimal outcome, and allocate scarce resources most effectively. Thus, both outcome and prognostic information are needed to treat and counsel patients and their families.

One tool to assess disease severity and to provide prognostic information is the APACHE II scoring system, which has three components: an acute physiology score, an age adjustment score, and a chronic health adjustment score. It remains commonly used because the instrument is supported by a large body of literature and allows comparisons to historical data. However,

Table 2. The Sequential Organ Failure Assessment (SOFA) scoring system.

FiO_2: fraction of inspired oxygen; MAP: mean arterial pressure; PaO_2: pressure of arterial O_2.
[a]Medication doses are given in mg/kg/min.

Variables	Scores				
	0	1	2	3	4
Respiratory PaO_2/FiO_2 (mm Hg)	>400	≤400	≤300	≤200	≤100
Coagulation Platelets (× 10^3/µL)	>150	≤150	≤100	≤50	≤20
Liver Bilirubin (mg/dL)	<1.2	1.2–1.9	2.0–5.9	6.0–11.9	>12.0
Cardiovascular[a] Hypotension	None	MAP <70 mm Hg no pressors	Dopamine <5 or dobutamine	Dopamine >5, epinephrine ≤0.1, norepinephrine ≤0.1	Dopamine ≥15, epinephrine >0.1, norepinephrine >0.1
Central nervous system Glasgow coma scale	15	13–14	10–12	6–9	<6
Renal Creatinine (mg/dL) or urine output (mL/day)	<1.2	1.2–1.9	2.0–3.4	3.5–4.9 <500	≥5.0 <200

Figure 3. Calculating the log odds of death for patients with acute renal failure.

BUN: blood urea nitrogen.

Log odds of death = 0.170(age) + 0.8605(male gender) + 0.0144(serum BUN) – 0.3309(serum creatinine) + 1.2242(hematologic failure) + 1.1183(liver failure) + 0.9637(respiratory failure) + 0.0119(heart rate) – 0.4432 × log(urine output) – 0.7207

the APACHE II scoring system has been criticized for lacking renal-specific criteria, such as serum urea nitrogen and oliguria, and for using the Glasgow coma scale, which is difficult to assess in mechanically ventilated patients. These shortcomings led to the development of the APACHE III scoring system, which has also been validated for critically ill patients with or without ARF [5,6].

Another scoring system, the Sequential Organ Failure Assessment (SOFA) system [7,8] (**Table 2**), was developed in order to better understand the progression of and interactions between failing organs (**Figure 1**). This tool was recently validated for ARF in a prospective, multicenter study using 1,411 patients admitted to the ICU [9]. The authors found that patients who developed ARF had a significantly higher mortality rate than other patients. Nonsurvivors were significantly more likely to have been oliguric and to have had more failing organs; the mortality rate was highest in patients with concomitant renal and cardiovascular failure.

In the hope of creating better prediction models, several renal-specific scoring systems have been developed. The most recent was developed by the PICARD Study Group [10], who performed a prospective, multicenter study to derive a model that can be used for all patients with ARF in the ICU. The model is described in **Figure 3**.

Table 3. Accuracy of general intensive care unit (ICU) and acute renal failure-specific prediction models.
APACHE: Acute Physiology and Chronic Health Evaluation; CCF: Cleveland Clinic Foundation;
PICARD: Project to Improve Care in Acute Renal Disease; ROC: receiver operation characteristic;
SAPS: Simplified Acute Physiology Score; SOFA: Sequential Organ Failure Assessment.

Prediction models		Area under ROC curve
General ICU models	APACHE II	0.634
	APACHE III	0.756
	SAPS II	0.766
	SOFA	0.756
Renal-specific models	Paganini (CCF)	0.718
	Liaño	0.630
	Schaefer	0.650
	PICARD	0.832

Accuracy of prognosis

Given the number of prediction models available, the primary question is how well they each perform. In the PICARD study [10], 605 consecutive patients with ARF in the ICU setting were assessed, and the capabilities of the various prediction models were compared. The area under the receiver operation characteristic (ROC) curve for each system is provided in **Table 3**. A model whose area under the ROC curve is close to 1.0 has a sensitivity and specificity approaching 100%, while a model whose area approaches 0.5 has no ability to discriminate, in this case, between survivors and nonsurvivors.

Several interesting and important conclusions can be drawn from these results. First, while the APACHE II scoring system is the most widely used tool to predict outcomes in ARF studies, it is perhaps the least accurate of all the available tools because it has the smallest area under the curve. The APACHE III scoring system performs better, which is not surprising given the increased number of renal parameters included in this instrument. Second, there is no overall difference in results when comparing the general intensive care scoring systems to the renal-specific scoring systems. This finding is somewhat disappointing given that these latter systems were specifically developed for ARF patients. However, the majority of these renal-specific scoring systems were developed at single institutions, which may explain their poor performance when applied to multi-institution studies. In contrast, the PICARD system was developed in a multicenter collaboration and proved to be the most accurate, at least in this one study. Finally, while these prediction systems may be useful in research studies, none of them is suitable for clinical application to individual patients. They unfortunately lack sufficient accuracy to be used as a basis for medical decisions and treatments. However, they may be useful in initiating or supplementing a discussion with patients and/or their families, especially as a deterioration of a patient's score over time is a strong indicator of worsening prognosis.

Conclusion

The outcome of critically ill patients with ARF remains poor. The data show quite clearly that developing ARF significantly increases mortality risk. However, this mortality risk is also dependent upon a number of factors – eg, the presence of MODS; for surgical patients, the type of surgery; and the requirement for renal replacement therapy. Over the last several decades, the mortality rate has fallen in these patients, presumably as a result of better understanding of the pathophysiology of these patients' illnesses and improved patient care. Unfortunately, none of the prognostic tools currently available allow the medical team or the patient's family to predict accurately the patient's survival or death. As a result, these models should not be the primary instrument used to limit treatment options or upon which to base medical decisions.

References

1. Chertow GM, Lazarus JM, Christiansen CL et al. Preoperative Renal Risk Stratification. *Circulation* 1997;95:878–84.
2. McCarthy JT. Prognosis of patients with acute renal failure in the intensive-care unit: a tale of two eras. *Mayo Clin Proc* 1996;71:117–26.
3. Biesenbach G, Zazgornik J, Kaiser W et al. Improvement in prognosis of patients with acute renal failure over a period of 15 years: an analysis of 710 cases in a dialysis center. *Am J Nephrol* 1992;12:319–25.
4. Druml W. Prognosis of acute renal failure 1975–1995. *Nephron* 1996;73:8–15.
5. Brivet FG, Kleinknecht DJ, Loirat P et al. Acute renal failure in intensive care units–causes, outcome, and prognostic factors of hospital mortality; a prospective, multicenter study. French Study Group on Acute Renal Failure. *Crit Care Med* 1996;24:192–8.
6. Chen YC, Hsu HH, Kao KC et al. Outcomes and APACHE II predictions for critically ill patients with acute renal failure requiring dialysis. *Ren Fail* 2001;23:61–70.
7. Vincent JL, Moreno R, Takala J et al. The SOFA (Sepsis-related Organ Failure Assessment) score to describe organ dysfunction/failure. On behalf of the Working Group on Sepsis-Related Problems of the European Society of Intensive Care Medicine. *Intensive Care Med* 1996;22:707–10.
8. Ferreira FL, Bota DP, Bross A et al. Serial evaluation of the SOFA score to predict outcome in critically ill patients. *JAMA* 2001;286:1754–8.
9. de Mendonca A, Vincent JL, Suter PM et al. Acute renal failure in the ICU: risk factors and outcome evaluated by the SOFA score. *Intensive Care Med* 2000;26:915–21.
10. Mehta RL, Pascual MT, Gruta CG et al. Refining predictive models in critically ill patients with acute renal failure. *J Am Soc Nephrol* 2002;13:1350–7.

Section 4

Renal replacement therapy

Part 1: Indications and modalities

Part 1: Indications and modalities

Michael A Kraus

Introduction

Acute renal failure (ARF) in the intensive care unit (ICU) requiring renal replacement therapy (RRT) occurs in 10%–30% of all ICU admissions in tertiary care hospitals. Unfortunately, medical management of ARF in the ICU has been disappointing. Medical support includes attempts to control and/or prevent volume overload and oliguria with fluid restriction and diuretics. While non-oliguric ARF has a better prognosis than oliguric ARF, the role and value of diuretics remain surprisingly controversial, with some data suggesting an adverse response. However, most clinicians still favor the use of diuretics to treat oliguria once the effective arterial blood volume (EAV) has been corrected. Other medical therapies used in the treatment of ARF include adjusting medications for the decrease in glomerular filtration rate (GFR) and avoidance of hypotension and other nephrotoxins.

When medical therapy fails, extracorporeal RRT is usually indicated. The ICU patient who requires RRT has significant morbidity and a high risk of mortality. Understanding the indications for RRT, how to prescribe therapy, and when to initiate therapy may improve outcome in these severely ill patients. This chapter reviews the indications for RRT, describes and compares the modalities available, and discusses some potential novel therapies in the ICU.

Indications for renal replacement therapy in the ICU

Historically, the indications for RRT in the ICU have been similar to those for the care of the patient with chronic kidney disease. While these indications for RRT are still valid today, newer and more aggressive therapies are aimed at improving mortality in these patients. Intensive and continuous therapies support the concept of improving the overall condition of the patient, thus allowing time for other therapies directed at the ICU patient's comorbidities to work. This overall care concept has been termed "renal support therapy" [1]. In other words, decisions regarding delivery of RRT in the ICU should be made with every effort to improve the patient's mortality risk and morbidity.

Indications for RRT can be simplified to the mnemonic "AEIOU" (see **Table 1**).

Acidosis

Historically, acidosis has been treated with RRT when caused by renal failure. As the GFR falls, acidosis typically worsens due to retention of organic acids and the inability of the distal tubule to secrete protons (and thereby generate bicarbonate). Initial treatment consists of bicarbonate replacement. However, this approach is limited by the potential for volume and

Table 1. Indications for renal replacement therapy (RRT): remember "AEIOU".
ASA: acetyl salicylic acid; CHF: congestive heart failure.

Acidosis	Electrolytes	Intoxications	Overload	Uremia
↓ HCO_3^-	↑ K^+	ASA	Nutrition	Altered mental status
↑ Lactate	↑ Na^+, ↓ Na^+	Theophylline	CHF	Pericarditis
↑ PCO_2	↑ Ca^{2+}	Lithium	Hypotension	Unexplained bleeding
	↑ Uric acid	Ethylene glycol		
	↑ PO_4^-, Mg^{2+}	Methanol		
		Cytoxan		

sodium overload. Thus RRT becomes necessary. Continuous RRTs have expanded this indication to include treatment of ongoing lactic acidosis or respiratory acidosis due to respiratory failure when ventilation cannot be improved.

Electrolytes

Electrolyte disorders can also be corrected by RRT. Any electrolyte abnormality can be improved by RRT, but hyperkalemia is the most common indication. As potassium rises above 6.0 mEq/L, the patient has an increased risk of fatal arrhythmias. Medical treatment includes intravenous administration of calcium to stabilize the myocardium and treatments to shift potassium intracellularly, eg, insulin, inhaled β-agonists, and $NaHCO_3$. Medications are then given to decrease the body's potassium burden, eg, diuretics and exchange resins (see **Section 2, Part 4**). Dialysis is indicated when hyperkalemia exists in the setting of renal failure, cell lysis, or rhabdomyolysis. In these states, hyperkalemia is difficult to control and likely to recur. Hypernatremia is usually treated with free water and hyponatremia with fluid restriction (see **Section 2, Part 2**). However, sodium disorders are very responsive to RRT and therapy is indicated when the disorder cannot be treated in the usual manner – usually when it is severe and associated with a depressed GFR. Uric acid, magnesium, calcium, and phosphorus disorders can be treated with RRT, particularly in the setting of ongoing cell lysis (tumor lysis syndrome) with renal failure.

Intoxications

Intoxications can also be treated with extracorporeal RRT. Dialysis can effectively remove intoxicants that have a low molecular weight, a low volume of distribution, and that are minimally protein bound. Hemodialysis has been shown to be effective for the treatment of drug intoxications due to aspirin (a level of >100 mg/dL), theophylline, lithium carbonate, cisplatin, cyclophosphamide, and high-risk barbiturate ingestion (usually in the setting of concomitant ethanol ingestion). Ingestion of ethylene glycol or methanol almost always requires dialysis to remove the alcohol, used in conjunction with ethanol or fomepizole (15 mg/kg intravenous load). High-flux hemodialysis is the most efficient form of extracorporeal RRT available in all intoxications, due to the high clearance of intoxicants. Peritoneal dialysis and continuous therapies can remove these substances but clearance is slower and less efficient.

Overload

Volume overload is treated with RRT when either oliguria or anuria exists. RRT is usually reserved for patients with oliguria unresponsive to diuretics. These patients are initiated on RRT when they have pulmonary edema, severe hypertension, or significant peripheral edema.

Uremia

Uremia is also an indication for RRT. Unfortunately, however, no clear definition of uremia in the ICU patient exists. Although clear uremic signs – such as mental status changes and pericarditis – are easily defined complications, they occur late in the course of disease and probably should not be used as markers for initiation of therapy.

Extracorporeal therapy for renal support in the ICU represents a change in focus from ameliorating the conditions directly resulting from lack of intrinsic renal function to supporting the patient and countering the effects of the complications arising from other organ failures. The goal of therapy becomes to increase survival time to allow for recovery of multiple organ systems as well as renal function. Potential indications for renal support are extensions of RRT and novel approaches for care in the ICU. Volume overload without oligoanuria or even significant azotemia is an indication for renal support. Continuous renal replacement therapy (CRRT) can be used in the patient with total body volume overload and less than adequate urine output despite a response to diuretics. Renal support can provide for nutrition, fluid removal in congestive heart failure, and total fluid management in the patient with multiple organ failure. Continuous therapies allow for continuous fluid removal in excess of inputs despite hypotension or pressor requirements. Postoperative mortality in the ICU rises as the fluid percentage of body weight increases [2] and CRRT may allow for this fluid removal postoperatively, thereby potentially reducing morbidity and mortality. Renal support also encompasses use of extracorporeal therapy in the setting of sepsis, congestive heart failure, permissive hypercapnia, and ongoing lactic acidosis.

Deciding when to initiate RRT in the ICU is a complex matter. Traditionally, waiting for a life-threatening indication for renal replacement has dictated timing. However, as we consider renal support needs and the extremely high mortality in these patients, earlier intervention seems warranted. Gettings and colleagues [3] retrospectively reviewed survival in trauma patients receiving CRRT in the ICU. In one group, CRRT was initiated early, when their blood urea nitrogen (BUN) was <60 mg/dL (mean 42 mg/dL); in the other group, CRRT was only initiated after the BUN exceeded 60 mg/dL (mean 96 mg/dL). Both groups received equivalent clearances and had similar characteristics; however, survival in the early group was 39% compared with only 20% in the late group [3].

In the absence of controlled trials, definitive guidelines on when to start RRT are not available. If the clinical approach to the patient in the ICU encompasses both renal support and renal replacement, then it is reasonable to initiate extracorporeal therapy when clinical experience suggests that an improvement can be obtained over the next 24 hours that outweighs the risk. Similarly, the decision to withhold RRT in the ICU should be based on the estimation that a lack of intervention with an extracorporeal therapy will not be

Table 2. Comparison of hemodialysis, continuous renal replacement therapy (CRRT), and peritoneal dialysis (PD).

cl/h: clearance obtained in an hour; cl/wk: clearance obtained over the course of a week; ICP: intracranial pressure; ICU: intensive care unit; IV: intravenous.

	Hemodialysis	CRRT	PD
Advantages	Efficient (cl/h) Dialysis nurse remains bedside More commonly performed Less cumbersome Short duration	Most efficient (cl/wk) Hemodynamically stable – Better tolerated – Provides stability Volume reduction, hence allows for IV input Bicarbonate administration 24-hour exposure No increase in ICP Designed for ICU needs	Hemodynamically stable Simple and inexpensive No anticoagulation required No increase in ICP
Disadvantages	Less efficient (cl/wk) Anticoagulation preferred May be poorly tolerated in the ICU setting Increases ICP Limited fluid removal Difficult to provide nutritional support	Anticoagulation preferred Excessive volume loss Cumbersome Requires ICU nursing training 24-hour exposure Filter losses Cost	Low clearances Infection risk PD access Respiratory embarrassment Potential to develop hyperglycemia Peritoneal leak

detrimental to the patient. In other words, if return of renal function is likely or if conservative management with furosemide, brain natriuretic peptide, or another pharmacologic therapy is likely to succeed without inducing further harm to the patient, it is reasonable to observe the patient without initiation of extracorporeal therapy.

Modalities of renal replacement therapy in the ICU

Peritoneal dialysis (PD), intermittent hemodialysis (IHD) (including daily), CRRT, and slow, low-efficiency daily dialysis (SLEDD) are all acceptable therapies in the ICU. The best modality has not been defined and each has its own advantages and disadvantages (see **Table 2**). CRRT offers recognized advantages in terms of continuous fluid and solute control but has never been convincingly shown to improve mortality. IHD can be performed in the ICU, and recent attention has been directed at increasing its frequency above the traditional thrice-weekly dialysis towards daily therapy. SLEDD increases volume control and small solute clearance above that obtained with IHD and approaching that of CRRT. PD is also used in the ICU but requires an intact peritoneal cavity. A decision regarding which modality to select is dependent on local preferences, cost, and availability of modality. However, ideally, the therapy should be tailored to the needs of the ICU patient. Regardless of the RRT utilized, the goal should always be to improve the patient's fluid, electrolyte, and acid–base balances, and allow for the greatest chance of renal and patient recovery.

Figure 1. Slow, continuous ultrafiltration.

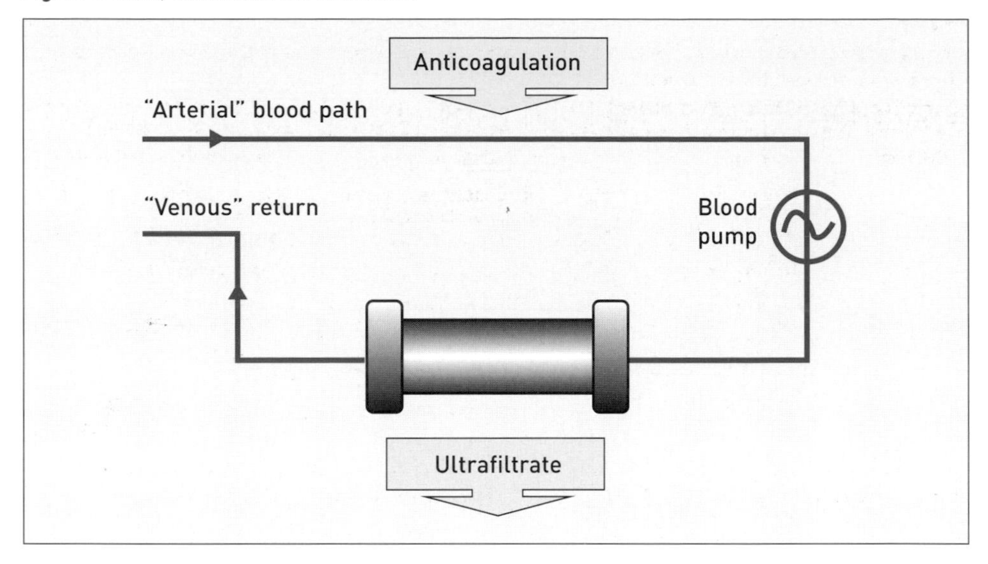

Continuous renal replacement therapies

Initially, continuous therapies utilized arteriovenous circuits. These were simple and inexpensive, but suffered from limited flow and clearance and required the placement of a large-bore arterial catheter, with attendant complications. The advent of reliable and easy-to-place double-lumen catheters heralded the development of continuous venovenous therapies. Venovenous therapy requires expensive and complex machinery but delivers reliable function without arterial puncture. Hence venovenous modalities have replaced arterial venous therapies.

CRRT can be performed in four basic modalities: Slow continuous ultrafiltration (SCUF); continuous venovenous hemofiltration (CVVH); continuous venovenous hemodialysis (CVVHD); and continuous venovenous hemodiafiltration (CVVHDF) (see **Figures 1–5**). Also see **Appendix III** for antibiotic dosing, **Appendix IV** for typical physician order sheets, and **Appendix V** for a typical CVVH flowsheet for the PRISMA system (Gambro Renal Products, Lakewood, CO, USA).

Slow, continuous ultrafiltration

SCUF is simply removal of fluid (desired hourly loss plus projected inputs) (**Figure 1**). SCUF is generally utilized in the absence of significant azotemia but with fluid overload ± fluid inputs at a greater rate than urine output.

Continuous venovenous hemofiltration

CRRT modalities designed for fluid and metabolic control require higher volumes of ultrafiltrate and hence require replacement fluid, dialysate fluid, or a combination of both. CVVH is an extracorporeal circuit with a double-lumen venous catheter hooked to an extracorporeal system with a blood pump, high-efficiency or high-flux dialysis membrane, and replacement fluid. As in SCUF, pure convection produces the ultrafiltrate; however,

Figure 2. Continuous venovenous hemofiltration – predilution.

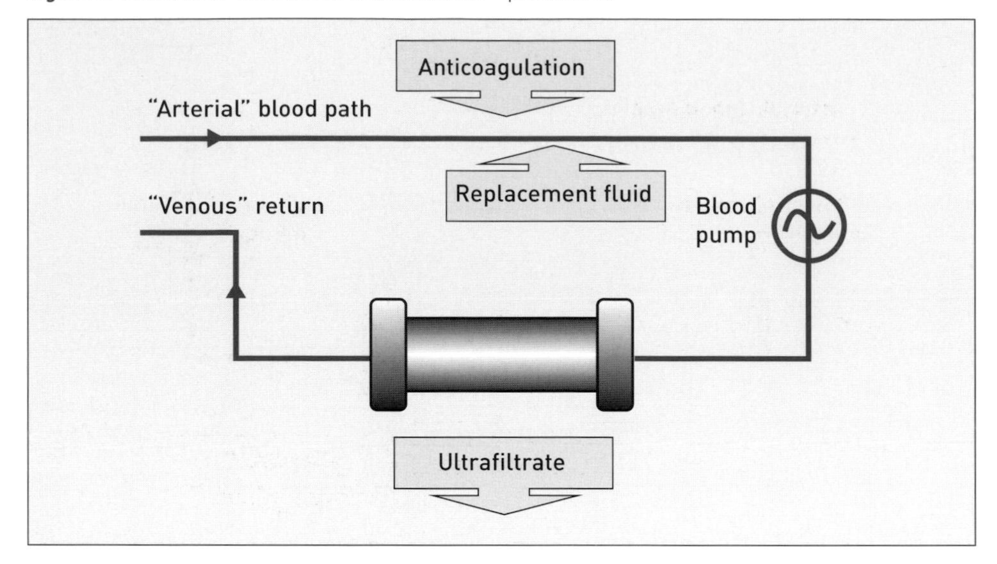

Figure 3. Continuous venovenous hemofiltration – postdilution.

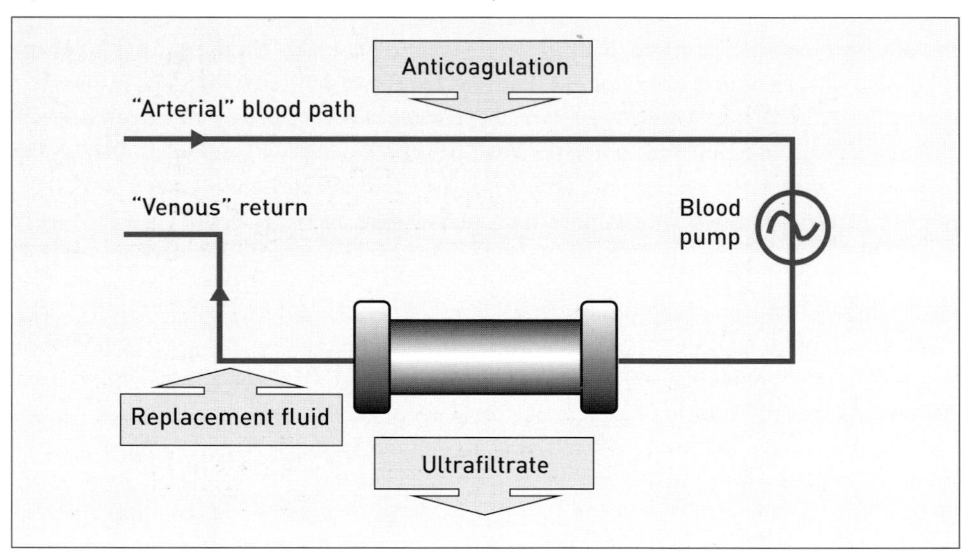

much greater volumes are generated. Volume status and metabolic improvements are maintained by the addition of replacement fluid in the circuit. Replacement fluid can be added pre- (**Figure 2**) or post-filter (**Figure 3**). Pre-filter replacement carries a benefit of less hemoconcentration within the dialysis membrane but decreases clearances by up to 15% [4]. Post-filter replacement maintains efficiency of the circuit but may be associated with an increase in thrombosis in the extracorporeal circuit. This latter point has been postulated but never demonstrated.

Figure 4. Continuous venovenous hemodialysis.

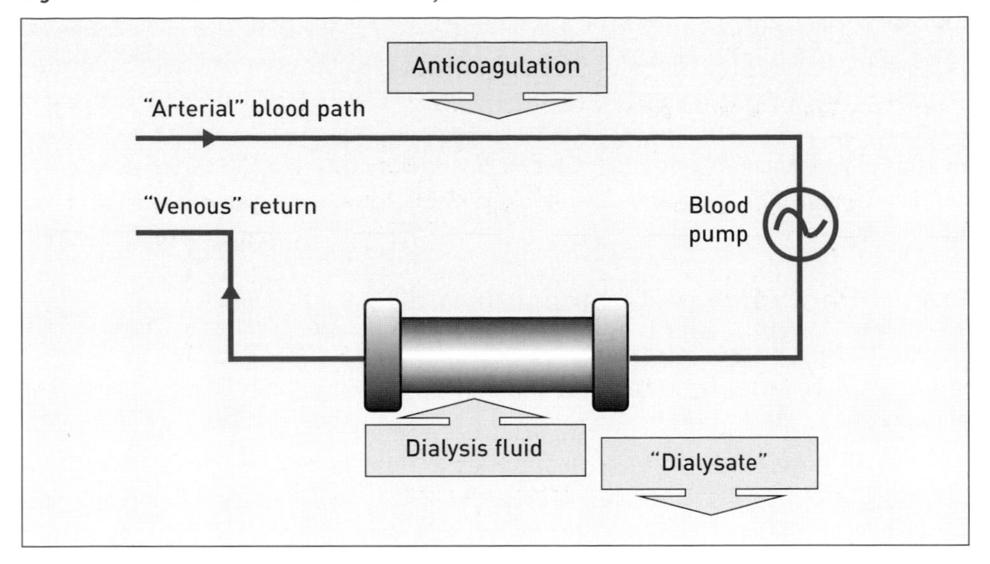

Figure 5. Continuous venovenous hemodiafiltration.

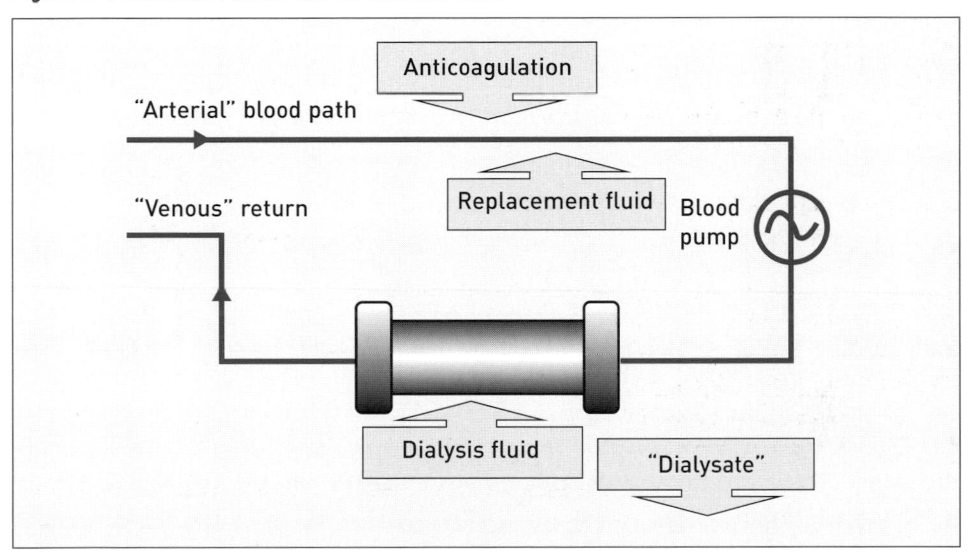

Continuous venovenous hemodialysis

CVVHD is an extracorporeal circuit with a double-lumen venous catheter hooked to an extracorporeal system with a blood pump, high-efficiency or high-flux dialysis membrane, and dialysate fluid (**Figure 4**). As in IHD, the dialysate runs countercurrent to the blood pathway. As in other forms of CRRT, low dialysis clearance is maintained by limiting dialysate volume to 1–3 L/h. While considered a diffusive therapy, convection may occur due to significant back-filtration.

Continuous venovenous hemodiafiltration

CVVHDF consists of an extracorporeal circuit with a double-lumen venous catheter hooked to an extracorporeal system with a blood pump, high-efficiency or high-flux dialysis membrane, and both replacement and dialysate fluid (**Figure 5**). In general, this combination is used to increase clearance with CRRT devices that have limited ability to raise replacement fluid or dialysate rates above 2 L/h. CVVHDF is also used to simplify citrate delivery for anticoagulation. Both diffusive and convective forces determine solute clearances in this form of therapy.

Intermittent renal replacement therapies

Conventional hemodialysis

Conventional hemodialysis is typically delivered in the ICU setting three to four times a week with a single-pool prescribed Kt/V (where K is dialysate flow, t is prescribed treatment time, and V is anthropometric volume) similar to that employed in patients with end-stage renal disease (ESRD). Recently, Schiffl and colleagues demonstrated improved mortality and renal recovery when the frequency was increased to daily [5]. Acute dialysis for ARF is typically performed with a high-flux or high-efficiency biocompatible membrane and is bicarbonate based. Conventional hemodialysis is diffusion based with ultrafiltration added as desired or tolerated to control fluid overload. Blood flow with intermittent therapies in the ICU ranges between 200 mL/min and 500 mL/min. It may be varied to reduce recirculation or to improve hemodynamic tolerance of therapy. Dialysate composition and flow are similar to those used in ESRD therapy, with dialysate flows of 500–800 mL/min. The duration of the therapy is typically 3–5 hours.

Slow, low-efficiency daily dialysis

SLEDD is a hybrid of continuous and intermittent therapies. Blood and dialysate flows are slowed to 200–300 mL/min and 100 mL/min, respectively, and therapy is prolonged to 8–12 h/day [6,7]. This slower form of dialysis theoretically allows for more hemodynamic stability with increased clearances when compared with conventional hemodialysis. SLEDD also allows for time off the extracorporeal circuit, allowing the patient to travel to diagnostic studies. Since SLEDD utilizes standard hemodialysis machinery, dialysate is generated online and the cost is potentially lower than that of CRRT, particularly if ICU personnel monitor the dialysis session, thereby obviating the need for dialysis nurses to be bedside for the 8–12 hours of therapy.

Peritoneal dialysis

PD can also be utilized in the ICU. An intact peritoneum is required and a temporary or permanent PD catheter is placed. Standard peritoneal dialysis solutions can be used. Clearance is convective and diffusive. Increasing the dextrose concentration in the dialysate and increasing the frequency of exchanges can adjust the degree of ultrafiltration. Transport kinetics are likely to vary between patients and have not been studied in the setting of ARF. Successful PD has been described in the ICU setting with adequate results [8]. However, PD has recently been demonstrated to be inferior to CRRT in the setting of ARF due to sepsis and malaria [9]. PD offers the advantages of a lack of need for anticoagulation, avoidance of vascular complications, and hemodynamic stability. Furthermore, it is performed with relatively inexpensive and simple systems. Disadvantages include the need for an intact peritoneum, potential development of hyperglycemia, potential respiratory embarrassment due to increased abdominal pressure, risk of peritonitis, and lower clearance than can be obtained with SLEDD or CRRT.

Prescription factors for renal replacement therapy in the ICU

Access

Access is an important feature in all forms of dialytic therapy. PD requires a peritoneal catheter; placement of a temporary catheter can easily be performed at the bedside. These catheters are firmer than standard catheters and are not cuffed or tunneled, hence temporary catheters are associated with increased catheter malfunction and an extremely high rate of peritonitis if the catheter remains in place for an extended period of time, particularly beyond 72 hours. Permanent cuffed catheters designed for use in ESRD can easily be placed in ARF. Bedside placement can be achieved using a modified Seldinger technique and a peel-away sheath, or with a peritoneoscope [10]. Alternatively, standard surgical placement by dissection or laparoscope can be performed in the operating room. The risk of peritoneal leak of dialysate is higher in acute PD, but the risk is acceptable.

Extracorporeal therapy requires adequate vascular access. Vascular access in the ICU is an important and overlooked aspect of extracorporeal therapy. Poor access can lead to significant recirculation and inadequate flows. Recirculation leads to less efficient therapy and delivery of less than prescribed clearances with IHD. Poor access flow rates and high recirculation are also detrimental in continuous therapies: hematocrit in the system rises, leading to clotting in the extracorporeal circuit. Adequate catheter function is probably the most important factor in maintaining filter patency. The factors that determine catheter function are the site of catheter placement and the location of the catheter tip.

Temporary non-cuffed, dual-lumen catheters are generally placed for use with RRT in the ICU. Most present-day non-cuffed dialysis catheters are manufactured using polyurethane. This is fairly firm for easy insertion but relaxes at body temperature. These catheters are placed via the Seldinger technique. Silicone catheters are thicker walled and more flexible. Placement requires a peel-away sheath or stiffening stylet. Non-cuffed catheters range in length from 13–24 cm. The 15-cm catheters are designed for placement via the right internal jugular vein. In most men and larger women, 19–20 cm may be required to reach the superior vena cava/right atrial junction. Larger catheters of >20 cm are designed for the left internal jugular and femoral approaches.

Cuffed catheters are designed for a tunneled placement. In general, these are placed when expected use of the catheter exceeds 2–3 weeks [11]. These catheters are silicone, hence are more flexible than acute catheters, and are longer. Placement is performed with a modified Seldinger technique using a peel-away sheath. Placement is more technically challenging. Cuffed hemodialysis catheters vary in length from 50–90 cm and are designed for internal jugular, femoral, trans-hepatic, or translumbar placement.

Dialysis catheters in the ICU should be placed in the internal jugular or femoral positions, with the right internal jugular usually preferred. Femoral catheter length should exceed 19 cm. The subclavian route allows excellent access when placed correctly but should be avoided whenever possible as subclavian catheter insertion is associated with an unacceptable rate of central vein thrombosis and stenosis [12]. Central vein thrombosis and stenosis leads to loss of potential sites for future arteriovenous fistulas and grafts. This is of particular concern as it is frequently difficult to determine which ARF patients might need chronic RRT either at the time of discharge or in the future. Despite this, a surprisingly high number of subclavian catheters are still used. According to the 2002 DOPPS study, 18% of European acute catheters and 46% of acute catheters in the USA were subclavian [13]. The characteristics of each site of catheter placement are listed in **Table 3**.

Care of the catheter

Catheter care is required to prevent malfunction and infection. Malfunction is usually related to thrombus or fibrin-sheath formation. Prevention with any particular type of locking solution is not proven. Most institutions continue to use heparin or 4% citrate as dictated by local policy. When catheter dysfunction is present, line reversal may be successful and is associated with acceptable recirculation.

Infection is prevented by use of excellent local care. Infection rates in acute catheters are minimized with the use of local antibiotic ointment with a dry gauze at the exit site [14]. Bacteremia is associated with the development of an exit-site infection and the duration of catheter use. For femoral catheters the risk of infection rises dramatically after 1 week, and the risk of internal jugular catheter-associated bacteremia rises after 3 weeks [15]: it is reasonable to try to limit catheter duration to within these periods. Once catheter exit-site infection is recognized, the catheter should be removed as the risk of bacteremia rises within days, even when treated – by 2% at 24 hours and 13% at 48 hours [15]. Catheter-associated bacteremia is treated with catheter removal and intravenous antibiotics [11].

Buffer

In PD, commercially available dialysates are generally used; the buffer in this solution is acetate. In intermittent dialysis and SLEDD, bicarbonate-based dialysate is generated in line.

Controversy exists over buffer selection for CRRT. Commercially-available dialysate solutions and peritoneal dialysate have been used as dialysate and replacement solutions, although these have only been approved for CVVHD. Peritoneal dialysate is hypertonic and not ideal. Commercially available dialysate solutions are either lactate- or bicarbonate-based; lactate-based solutions also contain calcium and magnesium. In lactate-based solutions, the lactate is converted to bicarbonate in the liver.

Bicarbonate base is preferred in patients with lactic acidosis or liver failure to prevent iatrogenic increases in serum lactate levels. However, even in patients without hepatic failure, systematic comparison of the two buffer systems tends to favor the use of bicarbonate – bicarbonate-based buffers are associated with lower lactate levels, less hypotension, better

Table 3. Properties of vascular access placement by anatomic site.

ICU: intensive care unit; IJ: intrajugular; SVC: superior vena cava.

	Femoral catheter	Internal jugular	Subclavian
Properties	Place for short-term use: <3 days in the bedridden patient	Preferred access when available, and patient can lie flat for placement	Should be avoided due to high incidence of central stenosis with use
Catheter length	Use >19 cm catheter: recirculation increases significantly with shorter catheters	13–17 cm on right 17–24 cm on left Place tip at junction of right atrium and SVC	13–17 cm on right 17–24 cm on left Place tip at junction of right atrium and SVC
Patient positioning for placement	Supine, lying flat if possible Knee mildly flexed, leg rotated and abducted	Patient in Trendelenburg position Face covered	Patient in Trendelenburg position Roll between scapulas Face covered
Complications of cannulation	Wire passing into an ileofemoral vein Puncture or damage to the femoral artery Retroperitoneal hemorrhage Increased infection	Puncture of the carotid artery Risk of pneumothorax, hemothorax Rupture of the SVC Pericardial tamponade IJ thrombosis	Puncture of subclavian artery Risk of pneumothorax, hemothorax Rupture of the SVC Pericardial tamponade Subclavian thrombosis (20%–50%)
Advantages	Safest approach "Least challenging" Can control bleeding Can place with patient semi-recumbent No pneumothorax risk	Low recirculation Lower lung injury than subclavian approach Low infection rate Low venous stenosis rate Ambulation possible	Low recirculation Ambulation easiest Low infection rate Patient comfort Easy to bandage
Disadvantages	Highest infection rate Non-ambulatory 1 week limit Recirculation highest	Technically difficult Carotid artery puncture Thoracic duct damage with left IJ approach Tracheostomy in way, and difficult to bandage in the ICU setting Trendelenburg position required for placement	Technically difficult Pneumothorax (1%–3%) Inadvertent arterial puncture Central stenosis rate Trendelenburg position required for placement

cardiovascular stability, and improved acid–base control [16,17]. Citrate is the main buffer/alkali utilized when citrate is used as an anticoagulant. Our institution favors the use of bicarbonate-containing solutions regardless of the modality of RRT used, whether CVVH, CVVHD, or CVVHDF.

Anticoagulation

RRT requires blood to circulate through an extracorporeal circuit, and hence maintenance of patency is required to deliver therapy. Clotting of the system leads to loss of blood, decreased delivery of therapy and/or decreased clearance, and increased costs of therapy. Patency can be affected by extracorporeal circuit design, catheter function, and anticoagulation delivery.

The extracorporeal system includes a blood pump, dialysis filter, air detector, and pressure sensors. By designing the system without drip chambers, no air–blood interface will be present. In addition, designing circuitry with lower resistance will allow for higher blood flows, which may lower the risk of thrombosis. Pre-filter replacement or fluid administration may reduce the risk of filter clotting. These changes in circuitry have all been hypothesized to improve patency of the system, but have never studied.

Experience indicates that catheter function is perhaps the most important element in maintaining patency of the circuit. Care must be taken to ensure proper placement and function. If a system has problems with recurrent thrombosis, changing the catheter frequently improves the situation regardless of the type of anticoagulation utilized.

The goal of anticoagulation is to improve circuit life and maximize the amount of replacement therapy that the patient receives; however, this goal needs to be balanced against the risk of bleeding and side effects. Tan and colleagues performed a prospective study comparing CVVH without heparin in "high-risk" subjects, and CVVH with heparin in the control group [18]. "High risk" was defined as ongoing bleeding, major hemorrhage within 48 hours, surgery within 24 hours, or international normalized ratio >2.0/partial thromboplastin time (PTT) >60 seconds. They found that the mean circuit life in the "high-risk" group was 32 hours compared with 19.5 hours in the heparin group. While they hypothesized that the "no heparin" group had a longer circuit life due to auto-anticoagulation, they concluded that CVVH without anticoagulation is feasible in patients at increased risk of bleeding. Generally, frequent saline flushes have been shown to be ineffective in increasing filter patency while adding increased manipulations of the CRRT system.

Anticoagulants, if desired, can be delivered systemically or regionally. Systemic modalities include standard heparinization to achieve a target PTT of 2–2.5 times normal (or activated clotting time of 70–90 seconds). Other systemic agents that can be used when heparin is contraindicated include prostacyclin, hirudin, and argatroban. Regional heparinization and citrate reduce the risk of bleeding complications compared with systemic regimens; however, they still pose an increased risk, and are difficult to use. In addition, citrate is associated with significant acid–base and electrolyte (calcium and sodium) disturbances. Because of potential complications, citrate therapy should only be used in centers familiar with its mode of action and its complications, and the center should be committed to frequent use of the drug (see **Tables 4** and **5**) [19,20].

A common problem in patients anticoagulated with heparin is the development of heparin-induced thrombocytopenia (HIT), an immune reaction usually mediated by anti-platelet factor 4 antibodies. Any further exposure to heparin will enhance the immune response. Additionally, there is 80% cross-reactivity between antibodies for heparin and low-molecular-weight heparins. Thus, any heparin or heparin derivative is contraindicated. Although there is no specific contraindication for the use of prostacyclin, the only US Food and Drug Administration-approved treatments for HIT are thrombin inhibitors. Several case reports have been published using lepirudin [21,22] and argatroban [23,24] in RRT. Because argatroban is hepatically eliminated, it is not renally dosed and has become the preferred thrombin inhibitor in these patients.

Table 4. Anticoagulation for the continuous renal replacement therapy circuit: heparin versus regional heparin.

ACT: activated clotting time; HIT: heparin-induced thrombocytopenia; PTT: partial thromboplastin time.

	Heparin	Regional heparin
Delivery system	Pre-pump heparin	Pre-pump heparin Protamine sulfate infused at venous limb of catheter
Monitor	System PTT or ACT	System PTT or ACT and patient PTT or ACT
Goals	PTT 70–90 s ACT 180–220 s	System: PTT >100 s (ACT >250 s) Patient: PTT 45 s
Advantages	Simple to use Easy to monitor No associated electrolyte acid–base disturbances	Regional anticoagulation Effective No associated electrolyte acid–base disturbances
Disadvantages	Highest risk of bleeding Risk of HIT	Risk of HIT Requires protamine More complex to monitor and adjust

Clearance

Recently, an increasing body of evidence has suggested that increasing the intensity and dose of RRT in ARF influences outcome [25]. Paganini and colleagues reviewed the outcomes of 844 patients with ARF requiring RRT in the ICU between 1988 and 1994 [26]. Although they found no difference in survival in the most or least severely ill patients, in those with an intermediate severity of illness score (the majority of patients) there was a significant improvement in survival at a higher rate of delivery of intermittent dialysis (Kt/V >1.0).

Schiffl and colleagues prospectively compared alternate-day to daily dialysis in the ICU [5]. They described a decrease in mortality from 46% to 28% in the patients who received daily dialysis versus the alternate-day group. They also described a reduction in sepsis and increased speed to recovery of renal function in the daily group.

Similarly, studies in CRRT also suggest a benefit to increasing the quantity of delivered therapy with increasing clearance rates. Storck and colleagues compared survival rates in a nonrandomized prospective study of continuous arterial venous hemofiltration (CAVH) and CVVH [27]. Survival was significantly higher in the CVVH group and correlated with increasing volumes of ultrafiltration delivered (7.5 L/day in the CAVH group and 15.5 L/day in the CVVH group). While Storck and colleagues compared two different techniques, the major difference in outcome and therapy was related to the quantity of therapy delivered, which is the main limitation of CAVH. No other technical factors appeared to affect survival.

More recently, Ronco and colleagues reported the results of a randomized study comparing the dose of therapy in CVVH [28]. Using a lactate-based post-filter CVVH system, they studied the differences in outcome in 420 ARF patients in the ICU randomized to receive replacement fluid rates of 20 mL/kg/h, 35 mL/kg/h, and 45 mL/kg/h. Delivered ultrafiltration rates were 31, 56, and 68 L/day. Survival was found to be significantly higher in the

Table 5. Anticoagulation for the continuous renal replacement therapy circuit: citrate delivery options.

ACT: activated clotting time; CVVH: continuous venovenous hemofiltration; CVVHD: continuous venovenous hemodialysis; CVVHDF: continuous venovenous hemodiafiltration.
Based on [19,20].

	4% Citrate	Citrate replacement solution
Delivery system	Pre-pump 4% citrate (150–200 mL/min) High-dose calcium administration systemically (8 g/L @ 40–45 mL/h)	Pre-filter replacement solution: - 145 mEq/L sodium - 1,106.5 mEq/L chloride - 140 mEq/L citrate - 11.5 mEq/L magnesium - 1,200 mg/dL glucose Rate of replacement: 1.5 L/h High-dose calcium administration systemically (20 g/L @ 50–70 mL/h)
Monitor	System ACT Patient ionized and total calcium Acid–base status	System ACT Patient ionized and total calcium Acid–base status
Mode	CVVHD or CVVHDF	CVVH
Advantages	No systemic anticoagulation Commercially available citrate	No systemic anticoagulation Isotonic delivery of citrate
Disadvantages	Low ionized calcium Elevated calcium gap Elevated anion gap Alkalosis Hypotonic dialysate – nonphysiologic solution Difficult to manipulate Requires expertise	Low ionized calcium Elevated calcium gap Elevated anion gap Alkalosis Limited clearance Difficult to manipulate Requires expertise
Other	Citrate delivery is based on blood flows of 100–150 mL/min and not for use with higher blood flows Citrate requirements and complications complications would rise at higher blood flows	Citrate delivery is based on blood flows of 100–150 mL/min and not for use with higher blood flows Citrate requirements and complications would rise at higher blood flows

35 mL/kg/h and 45 mL/kg/h groups (57% and 58%) when compared with the group of patients receiving 20 mL/kg/h (41%; $P<0.001$). Although not a primary endpoint, this study noted prolonged time to death with the higher therapies. In addition, BUN at time of initiation of therapy was significantly lower in survivors than in nonsurvivors.

Comparisons of modalities of RRT in ARF are few. Numerous retrospective and historical control studies have suggested that CRRT may be superior to IHD. However, few data comparing CRRT with IHD are available. Swartz compared CRRT and IHD in 349 ARF patients in the ICU at the University of Michigan, USA [29]. The study was not randomized and comorbidities were higher in the group receiving CRRT. After adjusting for comorbidities, no difference in survival was seen. Mehta and colleagues performed a prospective, randomized, multicenter trial comparing CRRT with IHD in 166 patients [30]. In this study, survival was found to be higher in the group receiving IHD (58.5% vs. 40.5%). However, the study excluded hemodynamically unstable patients and the randomization was flawed: patients in the CRRT group had significantly higher Acute Physiology and Chronic Health Evaluation (APACHE) III scores and a greater percentage had liver failure. Kellum and colleagues have attempted to reconcile these conflicting data in a meta-analysis of studies comparing CRRT and IHD [31]. Overall, there was no difference in therapy, but when low-quality studies were excluded, relative risk of death was shown to be substantially lower in patients receiving CRRT. However, the authors concluded that, given the overall quality of the studies reviewed, there was insufficient evidence on which to base strong conclusions.

While studies in the late 1970s and early 1980s purported to demonstrate the efficacy of PD over IHD, they were not randomized and do not reflect current methods of extracorporeal therapy. Phu and colleagues studied 70 adult patients with ARF due to either malaria (n=48) or sepsis (n=22) in Vietnam [9]. The patients receiving PD had a mortality rate of 47% compared with 15% in the CVVH group ($P<0.005$). The study suggests that PD is inferior to CVVH for treatment of ARF associated with malaria or sepsis.

Conclusion

ARF in the ICU requiring RRT is associated with significant mortality and morbidity. Over time, the etiology of death has changed from that due to complications of uremia to that due to complications of comorbidities. RRT needs to be prescribed based on the individual patient's needs, supporting the patient and allowing for time and other therapies to permit patient recovery. For the present, local preferences and expertise will continue to determine the delivery of RRT. In the future, the ability to achieve goals of toxin clearance, fluid stabilization, and control of electrolyte and acid–base derangements may dictate the type, frequency, and duration of extracorporeal therapies.

References

1. Mehta RL. Indications for dialysis in the ICU: renal replacement vs. renal support. *Blood Purif* 2001;19:227–32.
2. Lowell JA, Schifferdecker C, Driscoll DF et al. Postoperative fluid overload: not a benign problem. *Crit Care Med* 1990;18:728–33.
3. Gettings LG, Reynolds HN, Scalea T. Outcome in post-traumatic acute renal failure when continuous renal replacement therapy is applied early vs. late. *Intensive Care Med* 1999;25:805–13.
4. Brunet S, Leblanc M, Geadah D et al. Diffusive and convective solute clearances during continuous renal replacement therapy at various dialysate and ultrafiltration flow rates. *Am J Kidney Dis* 1999;34:486–92.
5. Schiffl H, Lang SM, Fischer R. Daily hemodialysis and the outcome of acute renal failure. *N Engl J Med* 2002;346:305–10.
6. Vanholder R, Van Biesen W, Lameire N. What is the renal replacement method of first choice for intensive care patients? *J Am Soc Nephrol* 2001;12(Suppl. 17):S40–3.
7. Marshall MR, Golper TA, Shaver MJ et al. Sustained low-efficiency dialysis for critically ill patients requiring renal replacement therapy. *Kidney Int* 2001;60:777–85.
8. Ash S. Peritoneal dialysis in acute renal failure in adults: The safe, effective, and low-cost modality. In: Ronco CBR, La Greca G, editors. *Blood Purification in Intensive Care*. Switzerland, Karger, 2001:210–21.
9. Phu NH, Hien TT, Mai NT et al. Hemofiltration and peritoneal dialysis in infection-associated acute renal failure in Vietnam. *N Engl J Med* 2002;347:895–902.
10. Kraus MA. Techniques of Peritoneal Dialysis Catheter Insertion. In: Gray R, Sands J, editors. *Dialysis Access: A Multidisciplinary Approach*. Philadelphia, PA: Lippincott, Williams and Wilkins, 2002:310–21.

11. III. NKF-K/DOQI Clinical Practice Guidelines for Vascular Access: update 2000. *Am J Kidney Dis* 2001;37(1 Suppl. 1):S137–81.

12. Cimochowski GE, Worley E, Rutherford WE et al. Superiority of the internal jugular over the subclavian access for temporary dialysis. *Nephron* 1990;54:154–61.

13. Pisoni RL, Young EW, Dykstra DM et al. Vascular access use in Europe and the United States: results from the DOPPS. *Kidney Int* 2002;61:305–16.

14. Oliver MJ, Edwards LJ, Treleaven DJ et al. Randomized study of temporary hemodialysis catheters. *Int J Artif Organs* 2002;25:40–4.

15. Oliver MJ, Callery SM, Thorpe KE et al. Risk of bacteremia from temporary hemodialysis catheters by site of insertion and duration of use: a prospective study. *Kidney Int* 2000;58:2543–5.

16. Zimmerman D, Cotman P, Ting R et al. Continuous veno-venous haemodialysis with a novel bicarbonate dialysis solution: prospective cross-over comparison with a lactate buffered solution. *Nephrol Dial Transplant* 1999;14:2387–91.

17. Barenbrock M, Hausberg M, Matzkies F et al. Effects of bicarbonate- and lactate-buffered replacement fluids on cardiovascular outcome in CVVH patients. *Kidney Int* 2000;58:1751–7.

18. Tan HK, Baldwin I, Bellomo R. Continuous veno-venous hemofiltration without anticoagulation in high-risk patients. *Intensive Care Med* 2000;26:1652–7.

19. Palsson R, Niles JL. Regional citrate anticoagulation in continuous venovenous hemofiltration in critically ill patients with a high risk of bleeding. *Kidney Int* 1999;55:1991–7.

20. Mehta RL, McDonald BR, Aguilar MM et al. Regional citrate anticoagulation for continuous arteriovenous hemodialysis in critically ill patients. *Kidney Int* 1990;38:976–81.

21. Fischer KG, van de Loo A, Bohler J. Recombinant hirudin (lepirudin) as anticoagulant in intensive care patients treated with continuous hemodialysis. *Kidney Int Suppl* 1999;72:S46–50.

22. Schneider T, Heuer B, Deller A et al. Continuous haemofiltration with r-hirudin (lepirudin) as anticoagulant in a patient with heparin induced thrombocytopenia (HIT II). *Wien Klin Wochenschr* 2000;112:552–5.

23. Kario K, Matsuo T, Yamada T et al. Increased tissue factor pathway inhibitor levels in uremic patients on regular hemodialysis. *Thromb Haemost* 1994;71:275–9.

24. Ohteki H, Furukawa K, Ohnishi H et al. Clinical experience of Argatroban for anticoagulation in cardiovascular surgery. *Jpn J Thorac Cardiovasc Surg* 2000;48:39–46.

25. Clark WR, Kraus MA. Dialysis in acute renal failure: is more better? *Int J Artif Organs* 2002;25:1119–22.

26. Paganini EP, Halstenberg WK, Goormastic M. Risk modeling in acute renal failure requiring dialysis: the introduction of a new model. *Clin Nephrol* 1996;46:206–11.

27. Storck M, Hartl WH, Zimmerer E et al. Comparison of pump-driven and spontaneous continuous haemofiltration in postoperative acute renal failure. *Lancet* 1991;337:452–5.

28. Ronco C, Bellomo R, Homel P et al. Effects of different doses in continuous veno-venous haemofiltration on outcomes of acute renal failure: a prospective randomised trial. *Lancet* 2000;356:26–30.

29. Swartz RD, Messana JM, Orzol S et al. Comparing continuous hemofiltration with hemodialysis in patients with severe acute renal failure. *Am J Kidney Dis* 1999;34:424–32.

30. Mehta RL, McDonald B, Gabbai FB et al. A randomized clinical trial of continuous versus intermittent dialysis for acute renal failure. *Kidney Int* 2001;60:1154–63.

31. Kellum JA, Angus DC, Johnson JP et al. Continuous versus intermittent renal replacement therapy: a meta-analysis. *Intensive Care Med* 2002;28:29–37.

Appendices

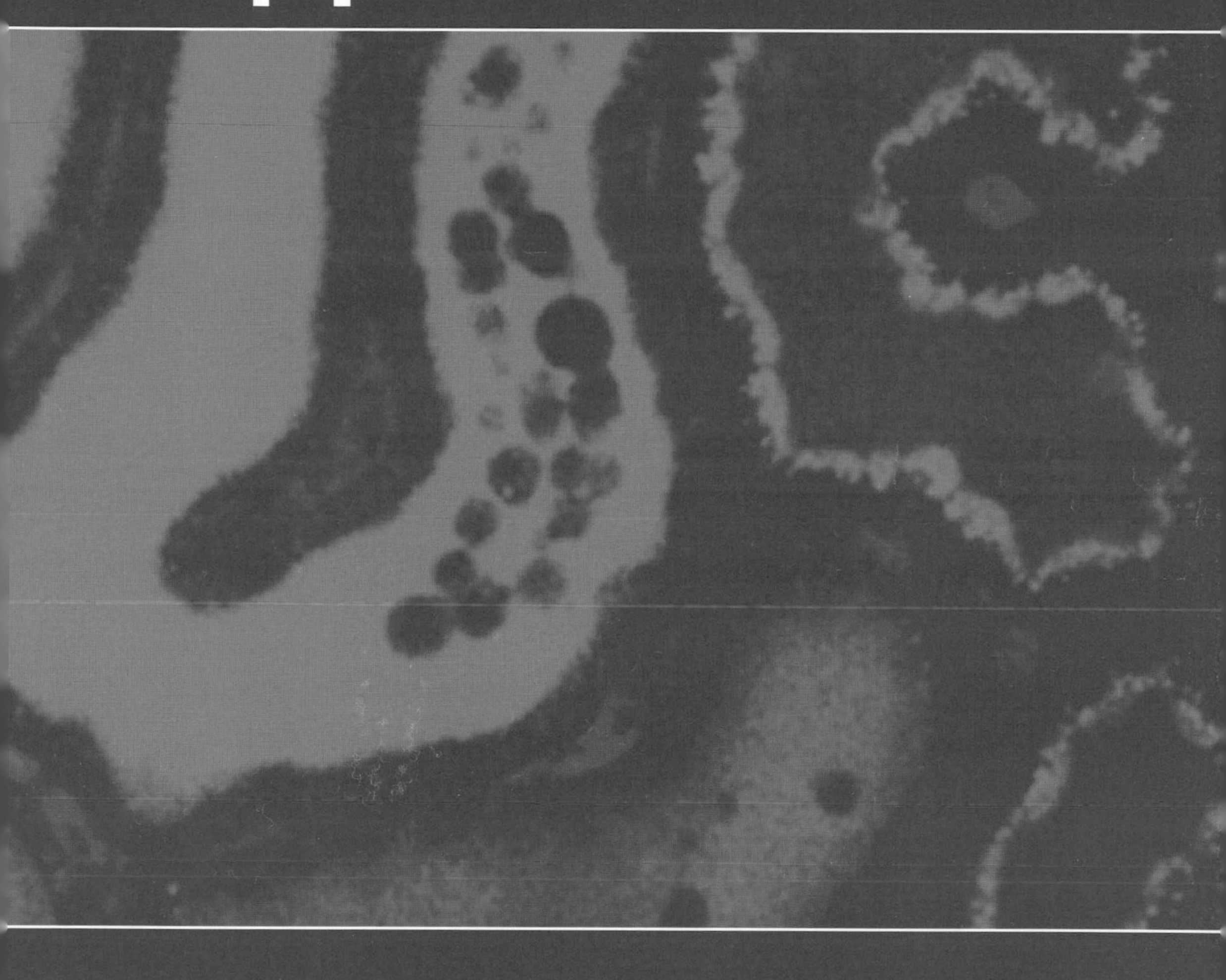

Appendix I. Hypernatremia example.

A 68-year-old man is found comatose and hyperthermic in a local sauna Physical examination – Weight: 70 kg – Pulse: 90 bpm – Respiratory rate: 20 breaths/min – Temperature: 39°C – Blood pressure: 130/80 mm Hg (supine); 110/50 mm Hg (seated) – Chest and cor within normal limits – No edema – Skin warm and dry with tenting
Laboratory results – Serum Na^+ 170 mEq/L – Urinary Na^+ 10 mEq/L – Blood urea nitrogen 30 mg/dL – Serum creatinine 1.8 mg/dL (normal: 1.2 mg/dL) – Glucose 100 mg/dL
Calculated water deficit: (0.4) × (70) × ([170/140] – 1) = (28) × (1.2 – 1) = 5.6 L Replace over 48 hours

Appendix II. Key issues in this case.

D5: 5% dextrose; I K^+: infusate potassium level; I Na^+: infusate sodium level; NS: normal saline; S Na^+: serum sodium level; TBW: total body water; Δ S Na^+: change in serum sodium per liter of infusate.

The patient is volume depleted. He has hypertonic dehydration and hypokalemia. He needs both volume and water. Increased insensible losses need to be anticipated due to fever.

$$\text{TBW} = (0.5) \times (70\ \text{kg}) = 35\ \text{L}$$

There are two ways to approach this case:

1. The patient can be given D5 0.45% NaCl with 20 mEq/L of KCl initially at 250 mL/h for 4 hours, then at 150 mL/h. A total of 4 liters of fluid will be given over 24 hours, with a calculated Δ S Na^+ of 2.03 mEq/L, or 8.12 mEq/4 L of D5 0.45% NaCl. A slow correction rate of 8–10 mEq/L/day is satisfied.

$$\Delta\ \text{S Na}^+ = \frac{(\text{I Na}^+ + \text{I K}^+) - \text{S Na}^+}{\text{TBW} + 1}$$

$$\Delta\ \text{S Na}^+ = \frac{(77 + 20) - 170}{36} = -2.03\ \text{mEq/L}$$

2. A second approach would be to re-establish volume with 0.9% NaCl (NS) at 250 mL/h for 4 hours, and then D5 water with 20 mEq/L KCl at 100 mL/h, for a total of 3 liters of fluid over 24 hours. The calculated rate of correction is 8.9 mEq over 24 hours.

   If NS with 20 mEq/L KCl:

$$\Delta\ \text{S Na}^+ = \frac{(154 + 0) - 170}{36} = -0.45\ \text{mEq/L}$$

   If D5 water with 20 mEq/L KCl:

$$\Delta\ \text{S Na}^+ = \frac{(0 + 20) - 170}{36} = -4.2\ \text{mEq/L}$$

Appendix III. Drug dosing in continuous renal replacement therapy (CRRT).

Doses need to be individualized for each patient. They assume normal hepatic function and anuria. If the CRRT system is discontinued, dosages should be adjusted to the patient's intrinsic renal function.

IV: intravenous; LD: loading dose; MD: maintenance dose; q: *quisque* (every/each);
SMZ/TMP: sulfamethoxazole-trimethoprim.

	CRRT replacement/dialysate solution rate (approximate creatinine clearance)				
Medications	1,000 mL/h (17 mL/min)	1,500 mL/h (25 mL/min)	2,000–2,500 mL/h (34–40 mL/min)	3,000 mL/h (50 mL/min)	>3,500 mL/h (>58 mL/min)
Acyclovir	5 mg/kg q 12 h	6 mg/kg q 12 h	10 mg/kg q 12 h	10 mg/kg q 12 h	5–10 mg/kg q 8 h
Amikacin	LD 10 mg/kg	LD 10 mg/kg	LD 10 mg/kg	LD 10 mg/kg	LD 10 mg/kg
Ampicillin	1 g q 8 h	1 g q 8 h	1–2 g q 6 h	1–2 g q 6 h	1–2 g q 4–6 h
Azithromycin	500 mg q 24 h	500 mg q 24 h	500 mg q 24 h	500 mg q 24 h	500 mg q 24 h
Aztreonam	1–2 g q 12 h	1–2 g q 12 h	1–2 g q 8 h	1–2 g q 8 h	1–2 g q 8 h
Cefazolin	1 g q 12 h	1 g q 12 h	1 g q 8 h	1 g q 8 h	1 g q 8 h
Cefepime	1–2 g q 24 h	1–2 g q 12 h	1–2 g q 12 h	1–2 g q 12 h	1–2 g q 8 h
Cefoperazone	1–2 g q 12 h	1–2 g q 12 h	1–2 g q 12 h	1–2 g q 12 h	1–2 g q 12 h
Cefotaxime	1 g q 12 h	1 g q 12 h	1–2 g q 8 h	1–2 g q 8 h	1–2 g q 6–8 h
Cefoxitin	1 g q 12 h	2 g q 12 h	1–2 g q 8 h	2 g q 8 h	1–2 g q 6 h
Ceftazidime	1 g q 24 h	1 g q 12 h	2 g q 12 h	2 g q 12 h	2 g q 8 h
Ceftriaxone	1 g q 24 h	1 g q 24 h	1 g q 24 h	1 g q 24 h	1 g q 24 h
Cefuroxime	750 mg q 12 h	1.5 g q 8 h	1.5 g q 8 h	1.5 g q 8 h	1.5 g q 8 h
Chloramphenicol	12.5 mg/kg q 6 h	12.5 mg/kg q 6 h	12.5 mg/kg q 6 h	12.5 mg/kg q 6 h	12.5 mg/kg q 6 h
Clarithromycin	250 mg q 12 h	250 mg q 12 h	500 mg q 12 h	500 mg q 12 h	500 mg q 12 h
Clindamycin	900 mg q 8 h	900 mg q 8 h	900 mg q 8 h	900 mg q 8 h	900 mg q 8 h
Famotidine (IV)	20 mg q 24 h	20 mg q 12 h	20 mg q 12 h	20 mg q 12 h	20 mg q 12 h
Fluconazole	200 mg q 24 h	400 mg q 24 h	400 mg q 24 h	400 mg q 24 h	400 mg q 24 h
Ganciclovir	2.5 mg/kg q 24 h	3 mg/kg q 24 h	3.5 mg/kg q 24 h	2.5 mg/kg q 12 h	2.5 mg/kg q 12 h
Gatifloxacin	LD 400 mg, MD 200 mg q 24 h	LD 400 mg, MD 200 mg q 24 h	LD 400 mg, MD 200 mg q 24 h	400 mg q 24 h	400 mg q 24 h
Gentamicin	LD 3 mg/kg	LD 3 mg/kg	LD 3 mg/kg	LD 3 mg/kg	LD 3 mg/kg
Imipenem	500 mg q 8 h	500 mg q 6 h	500 mg q 6 h	500 mg q 6 h	500 mg q 6 h
Levofloxacin	LD 500 mg, MD 250 mg q 48 h	LD 500 mg, MD 250 mg q 24 h	LD 500 mg, MD 250 mg q 24 h	500 mg q 24 h	500 mg 24 h
Linezolid	600 mg q 12 h	600 mg q 12 h	600 mg q 12 h	600 mg q 12 h	600 mg q 12 h
Meropenem	500 mg q 12 h	1 g q 12 h	1 g q 12 h	1 g q 12 h	1 g q 8 h
Metoclopramide	5 mg q 6 h	5 mg q 6 h	5 mg q 6 h	5 mg q 6 h	10 mg q 6 h
Metronidazole	500 mg q 8 h	500 mg q 8 h	500 mg q 6 h	500 mg q 6 h	500 mg q 6 h
Nafcillin	1–2 g q 4–6 h	1–2 g q 4–6 h	1–2 g q 4–6 h	1–2 g q 4–6 h	1–2 g q 4–6 h
Omeprazole	20 mg/day	20 mg/day	20 mg/day	20 mg/day	20 mg/day
Penicillin G	1–3 MU q 4–6 h	1–3 MU q 4–6 h	1–3 MU q 4–6 h	1–3 MU q 4–6 h	1–3 MU q 4–6 h
Piperacillin	4 g q 12 h	4 g q 8 h	4 g q 8 h	4 g q 6–8 h	4 g q 4–6 h
Procainamide	1.0 mg/min	1.0 mg/min	1.0 mg/min	1.0 mg/min	1.0 mg/min
Ranitidine (oral)	150 mg q 24 h	150 mg q 24 h	150 mg q 24 h	150 mg q 12 h	150 mg q 12 h
SMZ/TMP	5 mg/kg q 12 h	5 mg/kg q 12 h	5 mg/kg q 8 h	5 mg/kg q 8 h	5 mg/kg q 6 h
Synercid	7.5 mg/kg q 8 h	7.5 mg/kg q 8 h	7.5 mg/kg q 8 h	7.5 mg/kg q 8 h	7.5 mg/kg q 8 h
Timentin	2 g q 8 h	3.1 g q 8 h	3.1 g q 6 h	3.1 g q 6 h	3.1 g q 6 h
Tobramycin	LD 3 mg/kg	LD 3 mg/kg	LD 3 mg/kg	LD 3 mg/kg	LD 3 mg/kg
Unasyn	3 g q 12 h	3 g q 12 h	3 g q 6–8 h	3 g q 6 h	3 g q 6 h
Vancomycin	LD 15 mg/kg	LD 15 mg/kg	LD 15 mg/kg	LD 15 mg/kg	LD 15 mg/kg
Zosyn	2.25 g q 8 h	2.25 g q 6 h	2.25 g q 6 h	3.375 g q 6 h	3.375 g q 6 h

Appendix IV. Example orders with PRISMA (Gambro Renal Products, Lakewood, CO, USA) continuous renal replacement therapy.

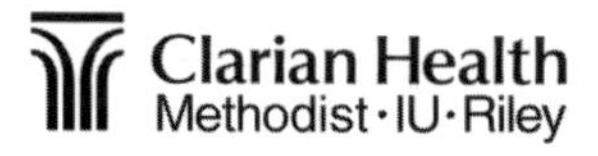

PHYSICIAN'S ORDERS

Initiate/Orders for PRISMA CRRT: CVVH CVVHD CVVHDF (Circle One) Page 1 of 2

Date	Time	
		1. **Admitting diagnosis**
		2. **Dialyzer –** AN69- M60 M100 set (Circle one)
		NO ACE INHIBITORS (while on CRRT)
		3. **Pt. weight** Q 12 h Q 24 h (Circle one)
		4. **Blood flow rate** ____________ mL/min (max. 180 mL/min)
		5. **Net hourly fluid loss**____________ mL/h
		6. **Set blood warmer temp**: 37°C 39°C 41°C None (Circle One)
		7. **Call** Renal Fellow/Nephrologist with lab results, Blood/Fluid orders, and any other questions
		8. **Labs**- CBC, Plts, A7 with A.M. labs and Q ___________hrs
		_____ ABG, Mg, PO_4, iCa^{++}, PTT, with A.M. labs and Q ___________hrs
		If Patient on Heparin/Protamine, draw system PTT and Patient PTT, Q ____ h and PRN
		9. **POCT** – ISTAT/BAM: pH, PCO_2, K, HCO_3, SO_2, TCO_2, Hb, BE, Creatinine
		POCT- ACT __________hrs
		10. **Replacement solution** ____________mL/h **Dialysate solution** __________mL/h
		11. **Standard fluid prescription**: 0.2% Dextrose 3 L
		KCl ______mEq/L (range 0-6 mEq/L)
		Na additives. Please circle one of the following:
		☐ **25 mEq/L Na Bicarbonate**, 115 mEq/L Na Chloride
		☐ **35 mEq/L Na Bicarbonate**, 105 mEq/L Na Chloride
		☐ **50 mEq/L Na Bicarbonate**, 90 mEq/L Na Chloride
		☐ **75 mEq/L Na Bicarbonate**, 65 mEq/L Na Chloride
		☐ **100 mEq/L Na Bicarbonate**, 40 mEq/L Na Chloride
		☐ **150 mEq/L Na Bicarbonate**
		12. OTHER DRIPS: (Stop continuous Ca/Mg IV infusions if filter goes down)
		☐ Magnesium sulfate 4 g/100mL water at _____ mL/h (Final conc. = 0.04 g/mL) ______
		☐ Magnesium sulfate 4 g/100 mL water over 4-6 h PRN Mg <1.5 mg/dL _____
		☐ Calcium gluconate 10 g/500 mL NS at _____mL/h (Final conc. – 0.017 g/mL, 0.075 mEq/mL)
		☐ Sodium phosphate 20 mm/100mL NS over 4 hours PRN PO_4 <2.5 mg/dL

MEDICAL RECORD COPY

CRRT PHYSICIAN'S ORDERS **T-5**

B-CLIN. NOTES	E-LAB	G-X-RAY	K-DIAGNOSTIC	M-SURGERY	Q-THERAPY	T-ORDERS	W-NURSING	Y-MISC

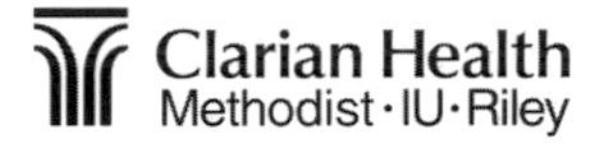

PHYSICIAN'S ORDERS

Initiate/Orders for PRISMA CRRT

Page 2 of 2

Date	Time	
		13. Anticoagulation via Prisma:
		☐ ______________ None
		Heparin 1000 units/mL (Drawn in 20 mL syringe on floor by RN)
		Heparin bolus: ________________units
		☐ A. Heparin infusion: __________________ units/h
		☐ B. Nurse heparin titration:
		Initial rate 10 units/kg/h
		Check PTT Q6h, titrate per below
		PTT — Bolus — Infusion
		≤42 s — 7.5 units/kg — ↑ 200 units/h (0.2 mL/h)
		43-54 s — 5 units/kg — ↑ 100 units/h (0.1 mL/h)
		55-75 s — None — No change
		76-100 s — None — ↓ 100 units/h (0.1 mL/h)
		>100 s — None — ↓ 200 units/h (0.2 mL/h)
		Call MD if 2 consecutive patient PTT >100 s or ≤42 s
		☐ Protamine 250 mg / 250 mL NS _________mg/h (Range = 5–20 mg/h) **Post Filter Only**
		Stop Protamine IV infusion if filter goes down

MEDICAL RECORD COPY

CRRT PHYSICIAN'S ORDERS

T-5

B-CLIN. NOTES	E-LAB	G-X-RAY	K-DIAGNOSTIC	M-SURGERY	Q-THERAPY	T-ORDERS	W-NURSING	Y-MISC
							■	

Appendix V. Example flowsheet designed for continuous renal replacement therapy with PRISMA (Gambro Renal Products, Lakewood, CO, USA).

PRISMA CRRT Flowsheet
Date ________________
Shift (circle): Day Evening Night
Therapy (circle): SCUF CVVH CVVHD CVVHDF
Pt Wt: 0400 _______kg 1600 _______kg
Prisma Serial #: ________________________________
PrismaTherm Serial #:________________________________

Clarian Health
Methodist · IU · Riley

Patient identification (DRAFT 3/03)

TIME												
RN initials												
Patient temperature												
Blood warmer temperature												
Heart rate												
Blood pressure												
A. Ordered net loss												
PRISMA Pressures (mmHg)												
Access												
Filter												
Effluent												
Return												
PRISMA Flow Rates												
Blood flow (mL/min)												
Heparin (units/h)												
Replacement fluid rate (mL/h)												
Dialysate fluid rate (mL/h)												
Non-PRISMA Intake (Projected h)												
B. Total												
Non-PRISMA Output (Previous h)												
C. Total												
Patient Fluid Removal Rate												
D. Rate (in increments of 10)												
Hourly Treatment History												
Replacement												
Dialysate												
Effluent												
Actual patient fluid removed												
Other IV Infusions												
Pressor name/dose												
Pressor name/dose												
Protamine dose												
Calcium dose												
Magnesium dose												

Initials/Signature:
____
____
____
____
____

8/12/24 I&O Calculation
Total non-PRISMA intake
– Total non-PRISMA output
– Actual fluid removed
= I & O Balance for time period

Calculation of Patient Fluid Removal Rate:
A Ordered Net Loss
B + Non-Prisma Intake Total
C – Non-Prisma Output Total
D = Pt. Fluid Removal Rate (set on Prisma)
Note: Pt. Fluid Removal Rate can only be set in increments of 10. Round up for all numbers not ending in 0.

MEDICAL RECORD COPY

PRISMA CONTINUOUS RENAL REPLACEMENT THERAPY (CRRT) FLOWSHEET

W-4

B-CLIN. NOTES	E-LAB	G-X-RAY	K-DIAGNOSTIC	M-SURGERY	Q-THERAPY	T-ORDERS	W-NURSING	Y-MISC

Abbreviations

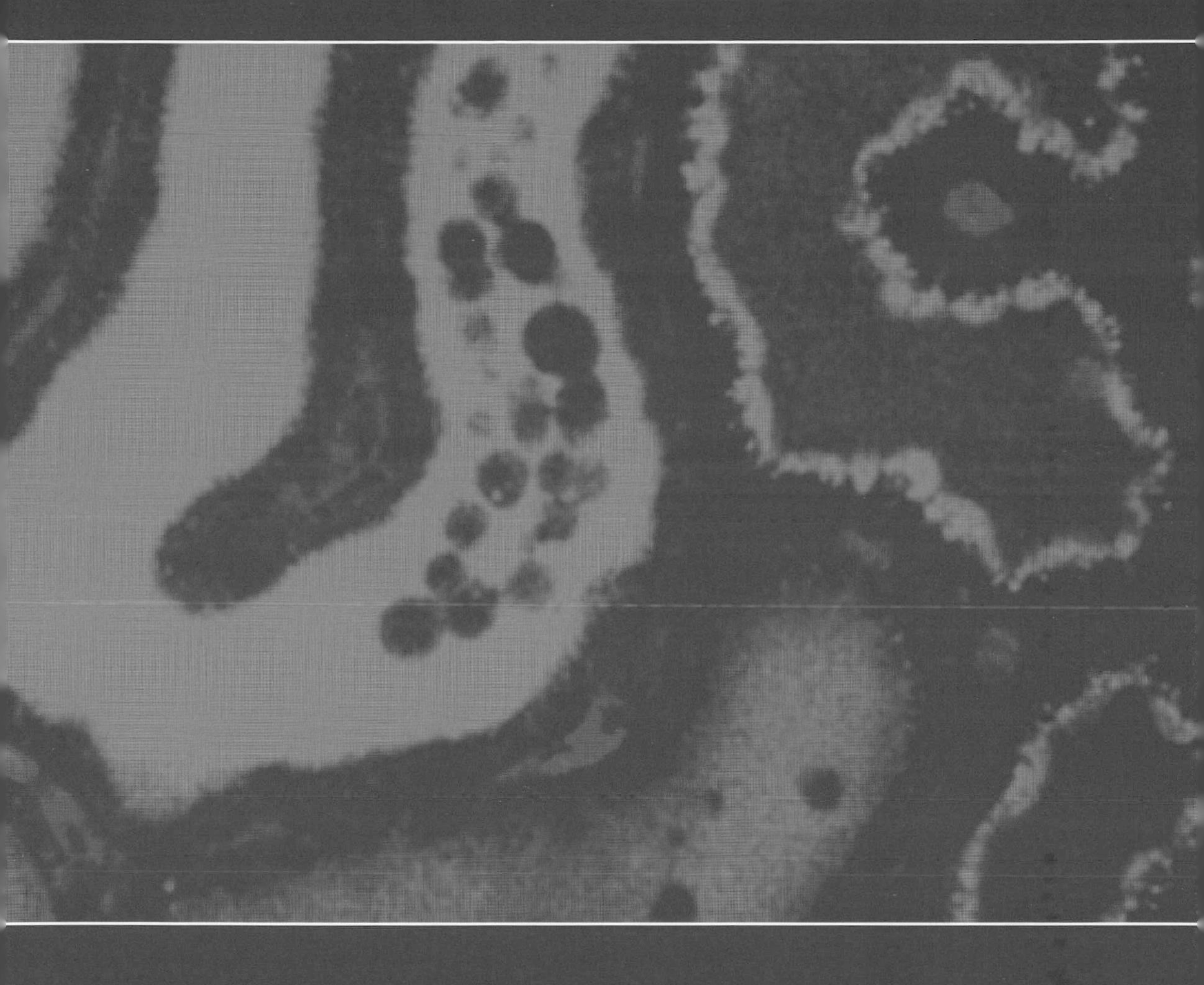

$1,2(OH)_2D_3$	1,25-dihydroxy-vitamin D_3
A	aldosterone
ABG	arterial blood gas
ACE	angiotensin-converting enzyme
ACT	activated clotting time
ACTH	adrenocorticotrophic hormone
ADH	antidiuretic hormone
AIN	acute interstitial nephritis
ALI	acute lung injury
APACHE	Acute Physiology and Chronic Health Evaluation
APC	activated protein C
AQP2	aquaporin-2
ARB	angiotensin receptor blocker
ARDS	acute respiratory distress syndrome
ARF	acute renal failure
ASA	acetyl salicylic acid
ATN	acute tubular necrosis
AV	arteriovenous
BCD	body chloride deficit
BiPAP	bi-level positive airway pressure
BNP	brain natriuretic peptide
BP	blood pressure
BS	breath sounds
BUN	blood urea nitrogen
CAVH	continuous arterial venous hemofiltration
CBC	complete blood count
CCD	cortical collecting duct
CCF	Cleveland Clinic Foundation
CHF	congestive heart failure
CKD	chronic kidney disease
cl/h	clearance obtained in an hour
cl/wk	clearance obtained in a week
CMV	continuous mandatory ventilation; cytomegalovirus
CNS	central nervous system
COPD	chronic obstructive pulmonary disease
COSM	calculated osmolality
CPAP	continuous positive airway pressure
Cr	creatinine
CrCl	creatinine clearance
CRF	chronic renal failure
CRRT	continuous renal replacement therapy
CT	computed tomography
CVVH	continuous venovenous hemofiltration
CVVHD	continuous venovenous hemodialysis

CVVHDF	continuous venovenous hemodiafiltration
D5W	5% dextrose in water
DHT	dihydrotachysterol
DI	diabetes insipidus
DIC	disseminated intravascular coagulation
DKA	diabetic ketoacidosis
2,3-DPG	2,3-diphosphoglycerate
DM	diabetes mellitus
DOC	deoxycorticosterone
EAV	effective arterial volume
EBV	Epstein–Barr virus
ECF	extracellular fluid
ECG	electrocardiogram
ER	emergency room
ESRD	end-stage renal disease
ETT	endotracheal tube
FBH	familial benign hypercalcemia
FE	fractional excretion
FEV_1	forced expiratory volume in 1 second
FiO_2	fraction of inspired O_2
FRC	functional residual capacity
GCS	Glasgow coma scale
GFR	glomerular filtration rate
GI	gastrointestinal
GN	glomerulonephritis
HELLP	hemolysis, elevated liver enzymes, and low platelets
HES	hydroxyethyl starch
HIT	heparin-induced thrombocytopenia
HPS	hepatorenal syndrome
HPTH	hyperparathyroidism
HSV	herpes simplex virus
HTN	hypertension
I	infusate
IABP	intra-aortic balloon pumping
IBW	ideal bodyweight
ICF	intracellular fluid
ICP	intracranial pressure
ICU	intensive care unit
Ig	immunoglobulin
IHD	intermittent hemodialysis
IL	interleukin
IM	intramuscular
IV	intravenous
LD	loading dose

MAP	mean arterial pressure
MD	maintenance dose
MDI	metered dose inhaler
MEN	multiple endocrine neoplasia
MI	myocardial infarction
MODS	multiple organ dysfunction syndrome
MOSM	measured osmolality
MRI	magnetic resonance imaging
MULEPAK	methanol, uremia, lactic acidosis, ethylene glycol, paraldehyde, aspirin, and ketosis
MV	minute ventilation
NE	norepinephrine
nebs	nebulizers
NG	nasogastric
NPO	*nil per os*; nil by mouth
NPPV	noninvasive positive pressure ventilation
NS	normal saline
NSAID	nonsteroidal anti-inflammatory drug
Ntg	nitroglycerin
NYHA	New York Heart Association
OD	overdose
ODS	osmotic demyelination syndrome
PaO_2	partial pressure of O_2 in arterial blood
pCO_2	partial pressure of CO_2
PCR	polymerase chain reaction
PCV	pressure control ventilation
PD	peritoneal dialysis
PE	physical examination
PEEP	positive end-expiratory pressure
PICARD	Project to Improve Care in Acute Renal Disease
PO	*per os*; orally
pO_2	partial pressure of O_2
prn	*pro re nata*; as needed
PS	pressure support
PSV	pressure support ventilation
PTH	parathyroid hormone
PTHrP	parathyroid hormone-related protein
PTLD	post-transplant lymphoproliferative disease
PTT	partial thromboplastin time
q	*quisque*; every/each
R	renin
RAS	renal artery stenosis
RBC	red blood cell
RBF	regional blood flow

RET	rearranged during transfection
ROC	receiver operation characteristic
RR	respiratory rate
RRT	renal replacement therapy
RSBI	rapid shallow breathing index
RSV	respiratory syncytial virus
RTA	renal tubular acidosis
S	serum
S Osm	serum osmolality
SAG	serum anion gap
SAPS	Simplified Acute Physiology Score
SBP	systolic blood pressure
SCUF	slow continuous ultrafiltration
SIADH	syndrome of inappropriate antidiuretic hormone secretion
SIMV	synchronized intermittent mandatory ventilation
SIRS	systemic inflammatory response syndrome
SLEDD	slow, low-efficiency daily dialysis
SMZ/TMP	sulfamethoxazole-trimethoprim
SOFA	Sequential Organ Failure Assessment
SPEP	serum protein electrophoresis
SVR	systemic vascular resistance
S_x	syndrome
TAL	thick ascending limb
TBW	total body water
THAM	tris-hydroxymethyl aminomethane
TIPS	transjugular intrahepatic portosystemic shunt
Tm	threshold/tubular maximum
TNF	tumor necrosis factor
TPN	total parenteral nutrition
TSH	thyroid-stimulating hormone
U	urinary
UA	urinalysis
UAG	urine anion gap
UN	urea nitrogen
USP	United States Pharmacopeia
USRDS	United States Renal Disease System
VSV	vesicular stomatitis virus
WBC	white blood cell

Index

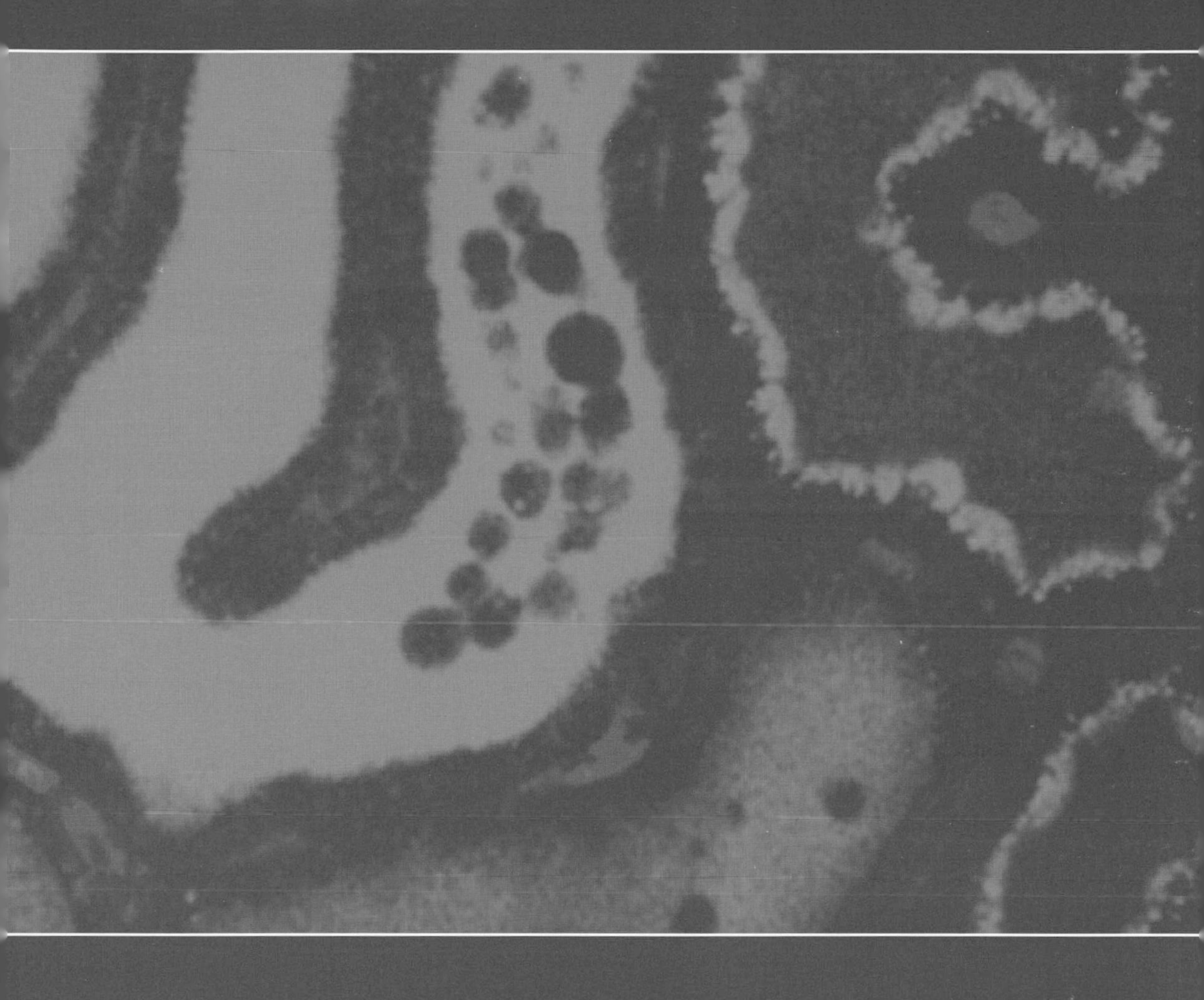

Page numbers in **bold** refer to figures.
Page numbers in *italics* refer to tables.
vs. indicates a comparison or differential diagnosis.